CELL NUTRITION

NEW SCIENCE OF HEALTH 100 FAQS

SACCHARIDES

Collected by
Lena Zheng Ph.D.

Copyright © 2015 Lena Zheng

All rights reserved.

Promoting Saccharides - Real Food Technology

ISBN-13: 978-1517303747

ISBN-10: 1517303745

祝福

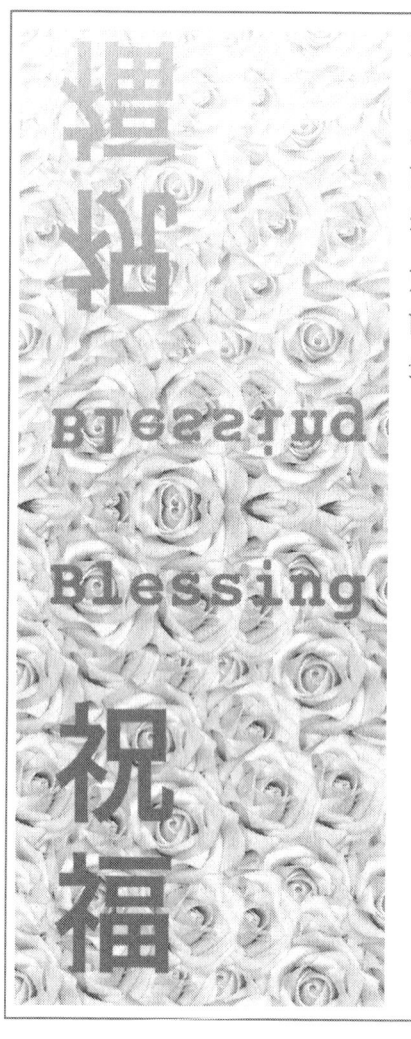

Blessing

Blessing

祝福

Dedicate this message straight from my heart to all who are striving to bring health, wealth, love in the whole world.

May hope, peace and joy be with you and your family.

愿一齐努力将从天而来的祝福佳音传给世界上追求健康富足关爱的人们。

From:

To:

PAGE

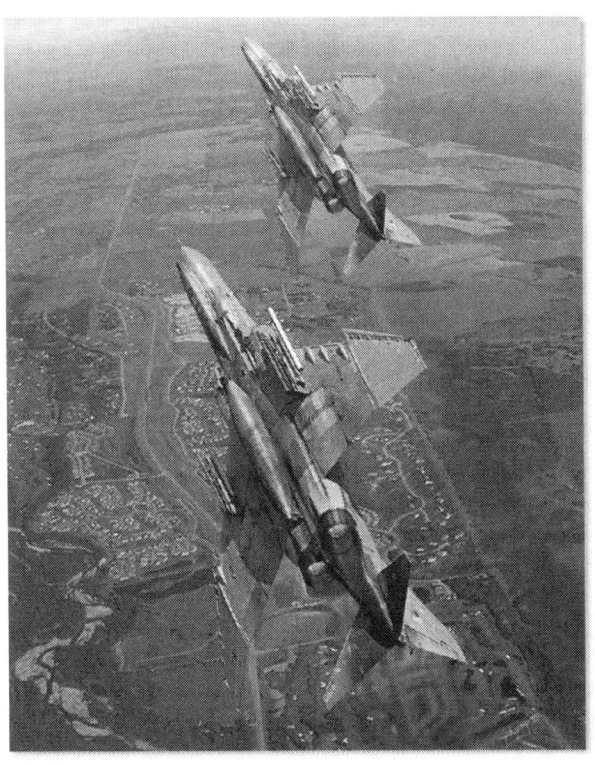

1 — **Chapter 1. Who Needs Saccharides?**
Every one needs Saccharides-the core of nutrition

5 — **Chapter 2. How do Saccharides Work?**
Magic effects of Saccharides in cells communication

14 — **Chapter 3. Which plants are used for Saccharides?**
Amazing health benefits of plants with Saccharides

20 — **Chapter 4. Why do people share Saccharides?**
Discovering of the science - Saccharides

30 — **Chapter 5. Where are Saccharides used for?**
Saccharides used for Health, Fitness & Skin Care

49 — **Chapter 6. What did Scientists & Doctors discover?**
Miracle effects of Saccharides in Immune System

CH 1. THE CORE OF NUTRIENTS - SACCHARIDES

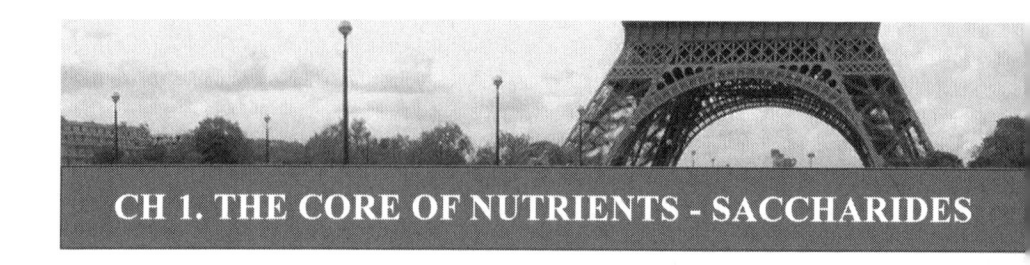

Every cell in our body - all 600 trillion of them - needs Saccharides .

What Does Our Body Need to function healthily?

In order to function healthily, our body needs Vitamins and Minerals* Fibre* Water* Essential Amino Acids* Essential Fatty Acids* Antioxidants* Essential Saccharides /Carbohydrates* . Daily exercise is very important. We also need to live in a non-toxic environment.

What are Saccharides ?

Saccharides are plant carbohydrates (monosaccharides). There are over 200 carbohydrates or sugars but only xylose* fucose* galactose* glucose* mannose* N-acetylglucosamine* N-acetylgalactosamine* N-acetylneuraminic acid (a sialic acid)* are essential to bodily function.

Why do Saccharides work as the key to a long, healthy life?

Science and medicine have long tried to understand the code by which the cells in the body communicate with one another in order for its complex functions to occur. For example, how does your digestive system know which food components to absorb into the blood stream and which to ignore? Or which cells to attack and destroy and which to protect and nurture? That code has now been broken. This role is undertaken by Saccharides . The most important discovery for your immune system in the last 100 years is something called Saccharides . Researchers proclaim it to be the most important discovery in the history of medicine - the key to a long, healthy life.

Why do Saccharides work as the key to effective cellular communication, proper cell function?

- Saccharides are the key to effective cellular communication and proper cell function. This has been established by the world's leading scientists and researchers. Saccharides are not vitamins, minerals, amino acids or enzymes, but are in a class of their own as nutritional supplements derived from plants.
- Glyconutritional supplements are formulated based on new understanding in the biochemistry of how the human body maintains health at the cellular level. Healthy cells lead to healthy tissue - healthy tissue leads to healthy organs - and healthy organs lead to healthy bodies.
- Medical doctors and the general public are becoming increasingly paid attention to the discovery of Saccharides , their functions, their importance in maintaining good health. Saccharides will soon become a part of standard care by medical practitioners for all auto-immune diseases, cancers, and degenerative diseases. A glyconutritional approach gets at the root cause rather than treating only the symptoms.
- Saccharides are however only part of what is necessary to a healthy body. Other important scientific discoveries of the past century highlight the importance of a range of other dietary or lifestyle factors including vitamins, minerals, fibre, water, essential fatty acids, essential amino acids, antioxidants, and exercise.

Who needs Saccharides ?

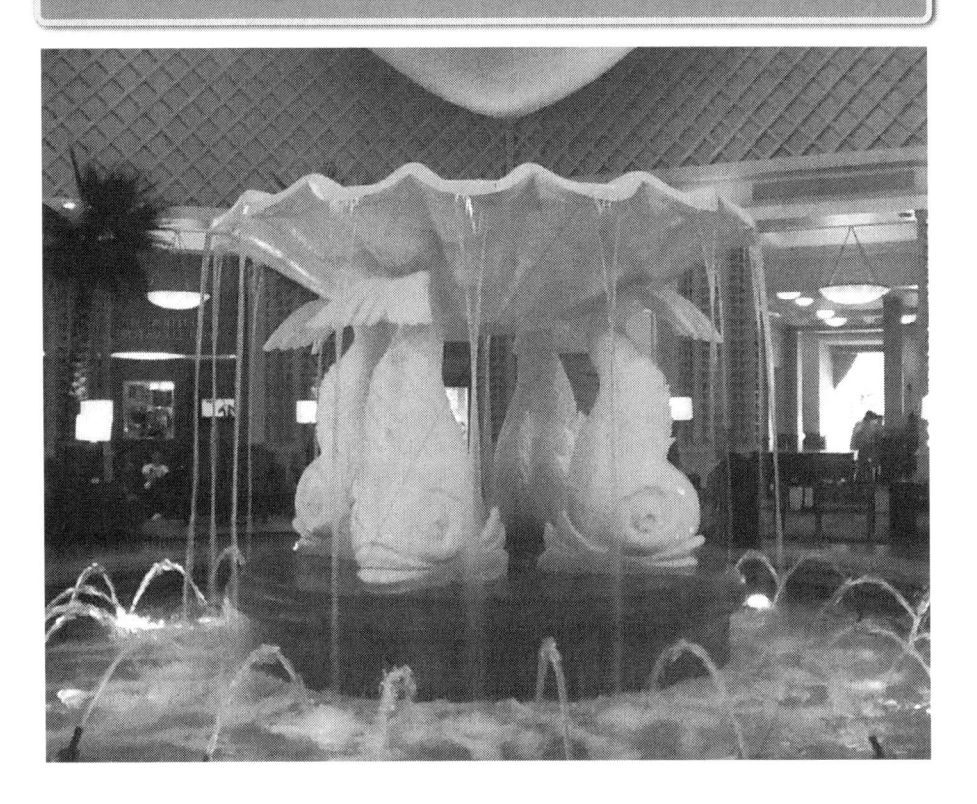

Healthy cells will make up healthy tissues, healthy tissues will then make up healthy organs, and healthy organs make up a healthy body. Through the cell-to-cell communication, our bodies find good cells in need of repair or nutrition, bad cells that need to be destroyed, and dead cells that need to be disposed. This process makes up a properly functioning immune system..

What is the carbohydrates therapy ?

The science at the heart of this discussion concerns carbohydrates molecules linked to most proteins and many fats in the body. These glycoproteins and glycolipids dot the surface of cells and serve as identification markers recognized by other cells. The field took off in the past 2 decades, and carbohydrates are now widely studied for their roles in normal biology and disease (Science, 23 March 2001, p. 2337).

How do Cells Communicate?

"Almost without exception, whenever two or or more living cells interact in a specific way, cell surface carbohydrates will be involved."

Bio/Technology
John Hodgson, 1990

Did scientists and doctors do lot of research and clinical testing?

Clinical testing soon began on mannose, the results were consistent and extremely eye-opening. However, there was one scientific issue, mannose was nothing more than a long chain carbohydrate (monosaccharides). Up to that time, all monosaccharides and carbohydrates were thought to provide energy at the cell level, and nothing more. But until now, scientists and doctors did lot of research in order to prove the idea that a monosaccharides molecule could help modulate the immune system.

What did scientists and doctors discover about cells communication?

The new technology became available that allowed scientists to look closer than ever before at the human cell In the late 1980's. It was discovered that on the surface of every cell are proteins, and connected to these proteins are tree-like structures of carbohydrate/monosaccharides molecules. It is through these tree-like structures that the cells in our bodies communicate to one another.

What are the technical difficulties to produce Saccharides supplement?

Stabilization keeps the monosaccharide molecule alive just like it was in the plant, which is the only way it will benefit the human body. Stabilization is very important because if not stabilized, these monosaccharides will start to die as soon as they are extracted from the plant.

Why has the term "Saccharides" become the latest buzzword in the food supplements arena?

The science of glyco-biology , the study of monosaccharides in relation to human health and disease, has remained a complex field addressed primarily within the domain of scientists, clinicians and health researchers.

How can we find the information about Saccharides?

The benefits of Saccharides are in a medical textbook called Harper's Illustrated Biochemistry from McGraw-Hill. Although the body can make other monosaccharides from glucose, "there is evidence that the other monosaccharides may be beneficial in some circumstances when added to the diet. This has led to the development of Saccharide supplements."

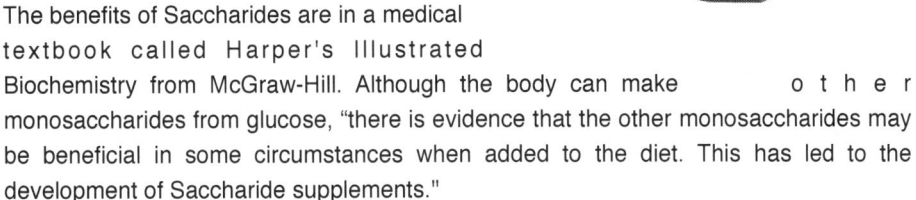

Why monosaccharides are important for Hunan body?

It is true that monosaccharides are not just "empty" calories but do, in fact, play an essential role in many biological functions, including cell-to-cell communication and immunity. There's actually an emerging and important field of science, called glycobiology, which explores the function of carbohydrates in health and disease. But Saccharide marketers have no basis for saying that consuming monosaccharides in supplements has health benefits. Enhances the immune system and treats a wide range of medical conditions, from diabetes and high cholesterol to psoriasis and multiple sclerosis.~ Berkeley university wellness news letter

Where can we find the Saccharide Research Published Reports?

Saccharides and their reportedly revolutionary effects on health when taken as nutritional supplements are being hailed in some quarters as the latest breakthrough in human nutrition and disease reversal. Published and presented papers on aloe vera active ingredient supported by research funding from Carrington Laboratories. The active principle isolated with immune modulating activity has been called, alcohol extracted freeze-dried aloe. There are 136 titles from 11 institutions produced by 55 investigators between 1987-1993. Search reports in Fisher Institute web pages.

CH2 The Magic effects of Saccharides

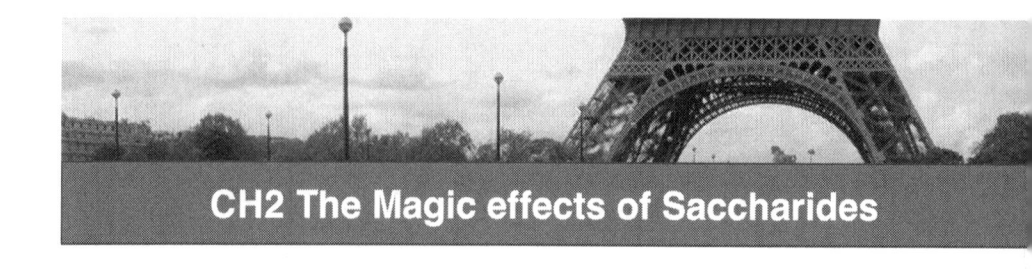

The Magic effects of Saccharides are specially in cells communication and Immune System.

What is the relationship between Saccharides and glycoproteins?

Saccharides are sugar molecules. 'Glyco' means sweet and so they are 'sweet nutrients'. The sugar molecules often form sugar chains known as glycans, and these chains of Saccharides then bind with protein molecules on protein strands to form glycoproteins. The process of forming glycoproteins is called glycosylation.

What is the relationship between Saccharides and Immune System?

The immune system is the body's way of defending itself against bacteria and other 'foreign' substances. The fundamental protective actions involve neutrophils, macrophages, killer cells, and T and B cells. The specific actions of these cells, and how Saccharides can support their function is explained below.

We often hear are immunodeficient and autoimmune, but what do they mean?

Immune dysfunction can result in the immune system being either overactive or underactive. An underactive immune system shows itself in such conditions as cancer and AIDS. If the immune system seems to be doing nothing to fight viruses, bacteria, and cancers it is called immunodeficient. Whatever the dysfunction, whether overactive or underactive, Saccharides have been shown to help, acting as immunomodulators.

Immunomodulators down-regulate the overactive system and up-regulate the underactive system. In fact, the Saccharides are not the primary immunomodulators - they cause the DNA and the cells themselves to immunomodulate.

On the other hand autoimmunity is the opposite of immunodeficiency and is evidenced in the body seemingly attacking itself as if it is confused as to how to respond. Autoimmune conditions can be either systemic or localised:

What are the Systemic Autoimmune Diseases?

Localised Autoimmune diseases, Rheumatoid arthritis (joints, less commonly lung, skin), Scleroderma (skin, intestine, less commonly lung). Coeliac disease, Crohn's disease, Ulcerative colitis (gastro-intestinal tract), Type 1 Diabetes Mellitus (pancreas islets), Lupus [Systemic Lupus Erythematosus] (skin, joints, kidneys, heart, brain, red blood cells, other), Hashimoto's thyroiditis, Graves' disease (thyroid), Sjogren's syndrome (salivary glands, tear glands, joints), Multiple sclerosis, Guillain-Barre syndrome (central nervous system), Goodpasture's syndrome (lungs, kidneys), Addison's disease (adrenal), Wegener's granulomatosis (sinuses, lungs, kidneys), Primary biliary sclerosis, Sclerosing cholangitis, Autoimmune hepatitis (liver), Polymyalgia Rheumatica (large muscle groups), Raynaud's phenomenon (fingers, toes, nose, ears), Temporal Arteritis / Giant Cell Arteritis (arteries of the head and neck), There is still some debate whether MS, chronic fatigue syndrome, and fibromyalgia are autoimmune conditions.

> Many of the sources of Saccharides, especially the essential Saccharides, have been used for centuries as healing medicinal compounds in many cultures around the world. The primary sources of Saccharides are fungi, saps, gums, and seeds, while the secondary sources are grains, fruit and vegetables. Information resource : Saccharides Reference website

How do Saccharides work?

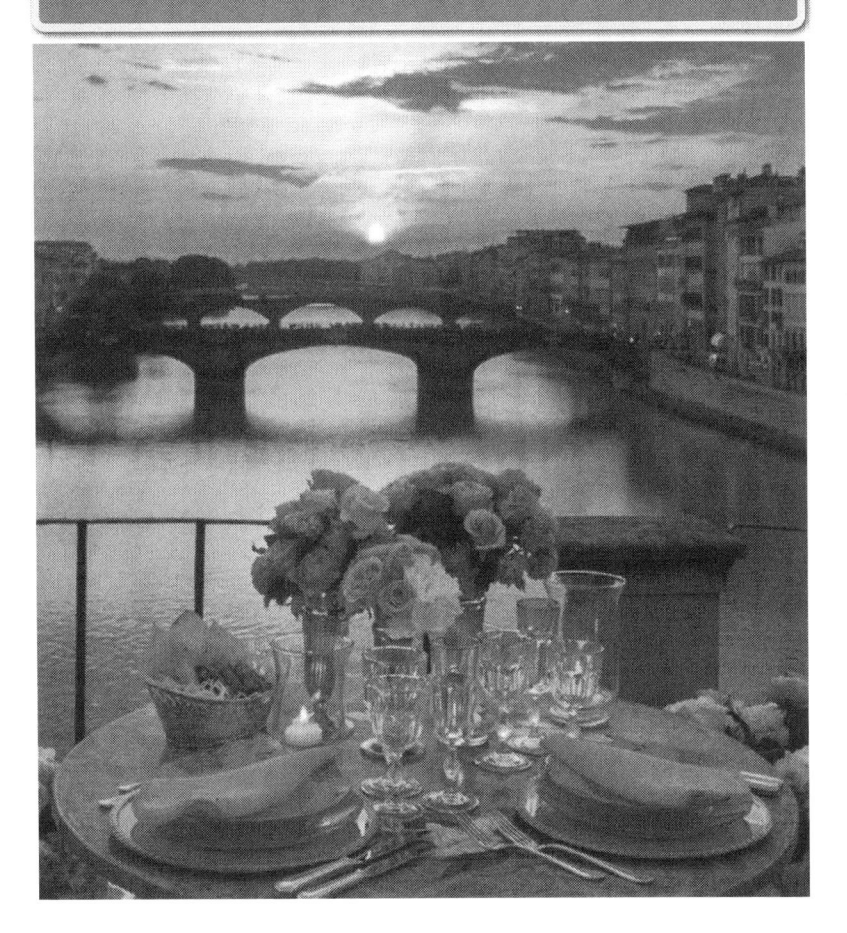

"Sugars That Heal."
by Emil I. Mondoa, M.D. & Mindy Kitei.

Glycoprotein Cell Receptors

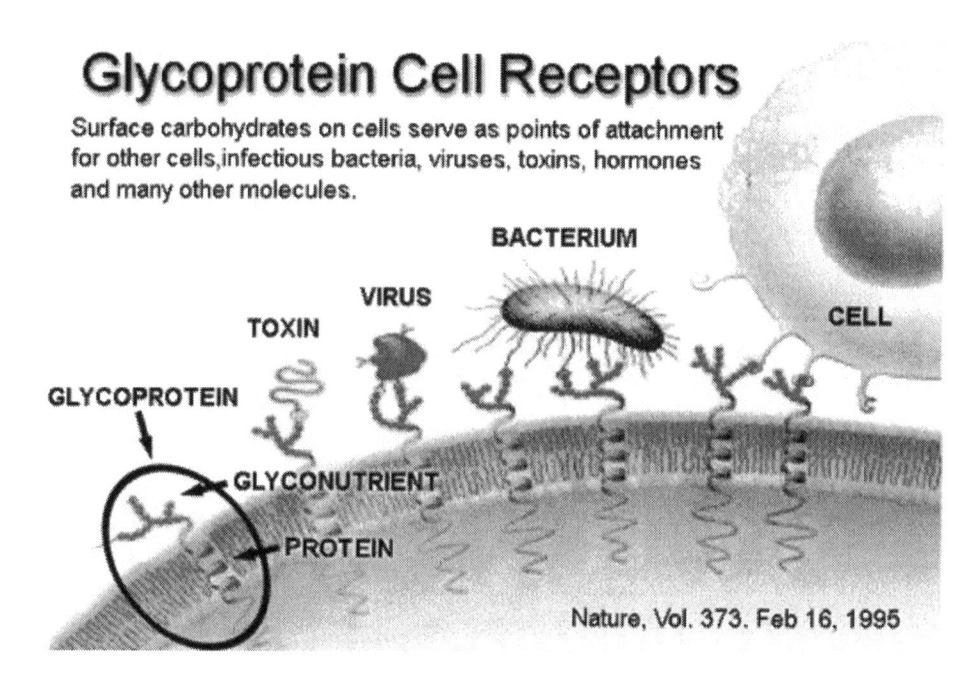

Surface carbohydrates on cells serve as points of attachment for other cells, infectious bacteria, viruses, toxins, hormones and many other molecules.

BACTERIUM
VIRUS
TOXIN
CELL
GLYCOPROTEIN
GLYCONUTRIENT
PROTEIN

Nature, Vol. 373. Feb 16, 1995

What are the meaning of Saccharides?
Glyco is a Greek word for sweet or sugar, naturally Saccharides are monosaccharides that provide a nutritional benefit. Saccharides are nutrients that your glyco needs to function properly. Saccharides are not vitamins or minerals. But just as there are essential vitamins, minerals, amino acids, and fatty acids, Saccharides are a newly discovered class of monosaccharides or carbohydrates that are also essential.

When you feel fatigue, well with Saccharides you feed your glyco some good with monosaccharides and in a matter of minutes, you are performing glycol-ectomies and glycol-summersaults once again.

Why is very difficult to get Saccharides in our body?
Saccharides refer to a finite group of essential monosaccharidess found among a pool of some 200 currently known types of monosaccharidess present in nature. The monosaccharides in Saccharides are not manufactured by the body and must be ingested via our food intake. In some cases, where there is a long term deficiency of these crucial monosaccharides, the body will attempt to synthesise them from glucose. However, this is an energy-sapping and inefficient process that requires 37 enzymatic

steps. Glycoproteins (Saccharides supplements) play a vital role in fundamental body functions at cellular level.

Which specific monosaccharides are important?
There are specific monosaccharides: xylose, fucose, galactose, glucose, mannose, N-acetylglucosamine, N-acetylgalactosamine, N-acetylneuraminic acid (a sialic acid).

How many kind of Saccharides do we get from our diet today?
The Saccharides are found in fruit and vegetables, but only in those harvested when fully ripe. This is concerning, considering that most of today's mass harvesting of fruit and vegetables takes place prior to the end stages of ripening. It's also clear from recent research that sectors of the population do not eat any kind of fruit or vegetable at all on a daily basis.

Saccharides contain monosaccharides obtained by plans. We just get two insteat of in today's diet because we no longer forage for our food off the land. Due to green harvesting, preservatives, and highly processed fast foods, we now need supplements of specific monosaccharides that make up Saccharides.

Why has lot of doctor never heard of Saccharides?
Most physicians attended medical school before this technology began being published so profusely. It wasn't until 1996 that one of the primary medical textbooks, Harper's Biochemistry, published a chapter on Saccharides. Although there are nearly 5,000 articles published dailypertaining to glycobiology, it is still not common knowledge. Physicians are inundated with new information primarily from pharmaceutical companies and this product being a neutraceutical, it is less known by today's doctors.

How do we get enough monosaccharides with emergency backup system?
Our body is a magic body, we have emergency backup system. Because it's essential for your body to have all specific monosaccharides, it was designed with the backup system to convert these specific monosaccharides from other carbohydrates. However, the backup system is not designed to be running continuously, and the process of converting just one of these monosaccharides is very complex and demanding because it requires many vitamin and trace elements that have also become deficient in our diets.

Why Saccharides are essential for maintaining optimal health?

> "Having recognized the tremendous potential of these monosaccharides, experts in the natural health field have already designed Saccharide supplements that are readily available to the consumer now."
> -"Miracle Sugars" Rita Elkins, M.H.

Inside your body, these specific monosaccharides provide the building blocks necessary to perform proper cell-to-cell communication. This cell-to-cell communication is your body's mechanism for maintaining optimal health. When it comes to healthy immune system function, these specific monosaccharides (Saccharides) are essential.

What are the role of Saccharides in cell health?
Saccharides play a crucial role in cell health. A healthy body is nothing more than a collection of healthy cells. Healthy cells make up healthy tissues, healthy tissues make up healthy organs, and healthy organs make up a healthy body. Saccharides link together to create a tree like structure called glycoforms. When glycoforms attach to a cell surface protein, they become glycoproteins. Glycoproteins and glycoforms cover the surface of a healthy cell. They can protect cells from infectious invaders, and are also responsible for the communication between cells and the rest of the body, including the immune system.

What are the Saccharide Supplements?
Saccharides supplement are the saccharides in certain plants get by real food technology. They are so important that our bodies have developed a backup process for producing seven of the essential Saccharides from one of the more readily available essential saccharides (glucose). This requires many bio-chemical steps, numerous enzymes, and can use up a lot of energy which may lead to fatigue. However, this process does not always complete successfully due to dietary problems, needed enzymes missing, environmental toxins, viruses, bacteria, etc. and, under stress, the body may not be able to manufacture enough of the essential monosaccharides.

Do Saccharides have side effects?
Because these are just food, they've not been found to have side effects or to interact with pharmaceuticals or herbal products kind of like eating broccoli. In fact, a physician is a last resort for children who have birth defects and childhood illnesses. She has been known to give these children very large amounts of Saccharides through feeding

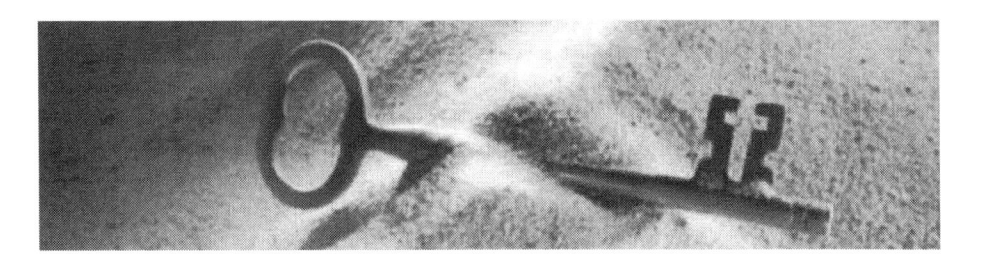

tubes with no side effects and very positive results. There lot of women get pregnant after using Saccharides.

How do Saccharides Work ?

The Saccharides are bound to a protein sting making them Glycoproteins, which is their final stage of development within the body. You may be surprised at the functions that Saccharides perform once they become Glycoproteins. They fill a structural role within the body in the form of Collagen, a transport role in Transferrin, Immunologic role in the form of immunoglobulin, cell to cell communication with selectins, proteins in fertilization, cell adhesion molecules, cell signaling by becoming receptors, clotting by becoming plasma proteins and lipoproteins, and lubrication in the body by becoming Mucins.

What are the medical research science results about Saccharides?

In recent years, great strides have been made in medical research science when it comes to cells, DNA, proteins and how these all interact with each other to produce results without our bodies. Research findings have also included things that appear when a lack of proteins or carbohydrates appears within the body. Saccharides are carbohydrates that have made their way into the research discovery arena. Saccharides are cellular identifiers. What they do is form a bank of terminals on a cell. These terminals are what everything else uses to attach to the cell. Everything else includes other cells, hormones, molecules as well as toxins, viruses and bacterium.

How dose our emergency back up systems work for getting specific monosaccharides?

When we don't get enough Saccharides in our diets and our emergency back up systems can't keep up due to stress, lack of proper nutrition, or even pollution, the glycoform structures are not properly created. Without the proper glycoforms, our

> "Many experts believe that immune system dysfunction is the greatest health threat we face. ...our immune systemshave been overworked and underpaid."
> "Miracle Sugars" - Rita Elkins, M.H.

bodies' cells become vulnerable and the communication process between the cells and immune system becomes broken, which can result in an over or under active immune system.

How dose our body react if we do not get enough specific monosaccharides?

As you can see from the examples Saccharides that form Glycoproteins, provide essential functions within the body. Without these carbohydrates or a sufficient amount of them within the body, there is nothing for the protein strands to bind to and so there is a lack throughout the entire body. The body is now forced to decide where these proteins are best used for survival alone. This can lead to a loss of healthy vital function within the body. If you think that, you might be lacking in Saccharides there are supplements available but please check with your doctor before starting them.

Why should Saccharides be viewed as immune system modulators?

we need our immune system to be balanced, an overactive immune system or an under active immune system, both are malfunctioned system. Saccharides should be viewed as immune system modulators that control cell to cell communication. They are critical in proper immune system function.

What is the surface cover of the healthy cell?

Saccharides are the basic building blocks that form glycoproteins, which cover the surface of every healthy cell. Cells communicate to one another via glycoproteins. Keeping your glycoprotein profile structures in the best possible shape by supplementing your diet with Saccharides, is the smartest and safest way to keep your immune system working optimally.

What is role of Immune system cells ?

Immune system cells are constantly roaming the body, going from cell to cell asking questions:
Do you (cells) need see, check, nutrition, restore, cleanse, destroy, protect or regulate? Depending on the response sent back, the immune cells will then:
1) Leave the cell alone 2) Send for help to repair, protect, or deliver nutrients to the cell
3) Call in the troops (killer cells) to kill and dispose of the foreign invader.

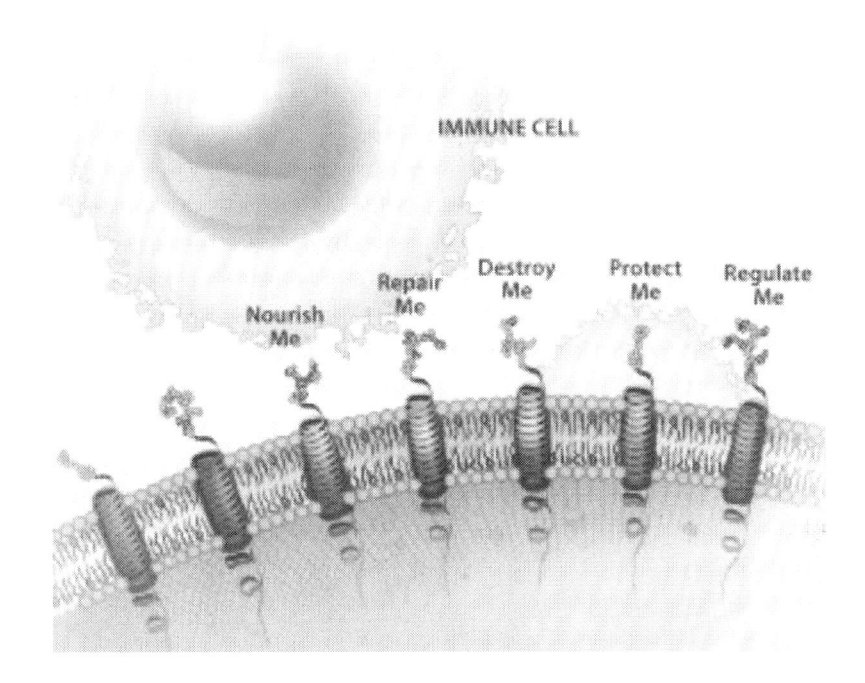

When does the communication between immune cells become broken?
The communication between immune cells can become broken when your glycoprotein structures are not properly developed because just one of these specific monosaccharides are missing. There are two cases:
•**An overactive immune system:** Immune system cells do some thing without asking and analyzing. The immune cells can become mis-guided and continually attack healthy cells and tissues.
•**Under active immune system:** Immune system cells do nothing even no asking. The dead or mutated cells can continue to proliferate without the immune system being called into action.

When one is missing, why dose the body have to manufacture it?
Multiple studies show the benefits of supplementing all specific monosaccharides, versus just one or two. When it comes to glycoprotein synthesis, all specific monosaccharides are required. If just one is missing, the body has to manufacture it. This is a long drawn out process, that steals energy and nutrition from the body, and keeps the immune system waiting before it can effectively do its job.

Some healthcare professionals consider your body to be in starvation mode when the emergency manufacture system is called into action. This system was not meant to be used on a regular basis. Not to mention the energy, vitamins and minerals needed to run the system are now also in short supply for most people.

How do Saccharides rebuilt the tissue of our body?
Saccharides transmit biologic information through cell to cell communication, Assist the formation of new tissue, particularly some types of collagen (the main protein of connective tissue) . They function in cell-signalling which is part of a complex system of communication that governs basic cellular activities and co-ordinates cell actions. Assist the body's immune function Are involved in hormone production.

How do Saccharides help the body to function normally ?
Saccharides help the body to function normally so that the body has a better chance of maintaining and healing itself naturally. Accurate communication between cells is vital for proper health and to synchronize many bodily functions. It is important to note that Saccharide supplements strength our cells, tissues, systems, body. They are not drugs and are not a cure or treatment for any particular illness. Taking Saccharides in our diets is a way of helping to maintain proper health and longevity.

Why have the "Saccharides" become the latest buzzword in the nutrients supplements market?
The study of Saccharides in relation to human health and disease, has remained a complex field addressed primarily within the domain of scientists, clinicians and health researchers in the science of glyco-biology field.

What is The role of Saccharides?
Saccharides are a breakthrough technology designed to deliver the vital missing ingredients not typically found in our diet: The human GI tract is something most people do not really think about, but it is something that plays a major role in how well the body functions.

Why is the important insight in the science study?
This study gives scientists insight into this complicated part of the human body and shows that Saccharides interact with bacteria in the digestive system. This study was accepted a couple of years ago for publication in The International Journal of Probiotics & Prebiotics. Its publication in this peer-reviewed.

CH3 AMAZING HEALTH BENEFITS OF SACCHARIDES

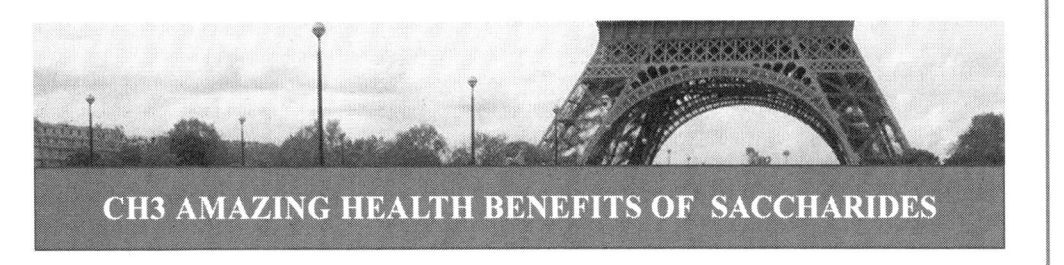

What are the Natural Sources of Saccharides ?

Aloe vera contains mannose, galactose and arabinose. The leaves are particularly rich in polysaccharides that provide healing and anti-infection properties when used both externally and internally. Aloe acts as an antifungal, antiviral, antibacterial, anti-allergy and antiinflammatory. It also protects the liver from chemical injury.

Mushrooms and fungi have been used medicinally in Japan and China for centuries with good results. They contain glucose, galactose and mannose which are known immune system boosters. They have anti-tumour actions, suppress inappropriate immune reactions, and act as modulators of the immune system.

Mushrooms contain a polysaccharide containing beta-glucans, called lentinant, which stimulates the white blood cells to devour invaders and detoxify or clean up the toxins they leave behind. The beta-glucans have been shown to fight cancer and tumour growth thus extending cancer survival time, fight infection in people who have suffered traumatic injuries and protect people from going into shock from severe infections, improve recovery from radiation treatments, and boost wound healing.

Saps and gums : Gum acacia from the African acacia tree contains galactose, rhamnose, arabinose, and glucuronic acid. Gum acacia has been shown to promote healing of irritated gastrointestinal mucosa and respiratory tract tissue, improve beneficial intestinal flora, control colon bifidus fermentation, and lowers triglyceride production, and serum cholesterol.

Gum ghatti from the gum of the Indian sumac contains galactose, arabinose, mannose, xylose, and glucuronic acid. The three essential Saccharides in this gum are important for cell-cell communication and lowering cholesterol. This gum is also beneficial for bifidus fermentation.

Latrix deciduai or larch tree contains arabinogalactan. Arabinogalactan studies show it has an anti-inflammatory and anti-allergic benefit. It also has been shown to block liver lectins what mediate tumour metastisis; block settling sarcoma L01 tumour ells, and protects intestinal mucosa against disease ad cancer promoting agents. Arabinogalactan also aids recovery from chronic fatigue syndrome.

The Saccharides in the stem and branches of Astragalus gummifer are galactose, arabinose, xylose, fucose, rhamnose, and galcturonic acid. The benefits include action as an antioxidant, diuretic, anti-inflammatory. It inhibits tumour growth, offsets the immune suppression of cancer chemotherapy. Astragalus gummifer also stimulates synthesis of antibodies, delays the natural aging process of blastocysts (fertilised egg cells) by one third, increases the number of stem cells in marrow and lymph and stimulates stem cell development into active immune cells.

Seaweed - Undaria pinnatifida

Undaria pinnatifida, a brown macro seaweed, is one of the richest known sources of in fucose. Fucose influences brain development (fucose is found in human breast milk); acts as an immune modulator; inhibits tumour growth and its spread; and enhances cell-cell communication. High concentrations of fucose are found at the junctions between nerves, in the kidney and testes and in the outer layer of the skin.

Echinacea contains arabinogalactan and galactose and has the benefits gained from the intake of these Saccharides .

Why are our diets deficient in Saccharides ?

The so-called fresh fruits and vegetables we buy today have few Saccharides (or nutritional value at all) because they are often grown in nutrient-deficient soil, picked before they ripen naturally, gassed, irradiated, artificially ripened, stored for days, weeks, or months, cooked, frozen, canned, processed, refined, pasteurised, genetically engineered, etc. Cooking and processing deplete Saccharides further.

Glycobiology has also found that beneficial bacteria in the colon breakdown polysaccharides to monosaccharides (Saccharides). But the bacterial content of modern people is different from our ancestors and so this process is less efficient.

Green harvesting allows long distance transport and allows fruit and vegetables to be stored for lengthy periods, but most of the essential Saccharides are found only in food that is ripened on the vine/tree and they remain in the fruit or vegetable for only 48 hours after picking.

Consider the tomato: Green harvesting loses up to 25% of its nutrients, Transporting loses up to 25% of its remaining nutrients, Storage loses up to 50% of its remaining nutrients, Canning loses up to 83% of its remaining nutrients, Cooking loses up to 50% of its remaining nutrients.

This leaves the tomato with 2.39% of it original nutrient content.

At the same time that our food has been reducing in nutrients, autoimmune diseases, cardiovascular disease, cancer, diabetes and chronic degenerative disease have been increasing alarmingly and have been occurring in younger age groups.

A growing mountain of evidence shows that all these diseases are caused by a single dietary deficiency: Saccharides that are missing from our diet. A dietary deficiency cannot be corrected with drugs or anything else, other than the missing nutrients. Amongst the missing nutrients in our food today are the antioxidants which help to control free radicals and support our body to deal with environmental toxins. Learn more about toxins and free radicals.

Being proactive and taking control of our wellness by seeking to ensure that our body has the essential ingredients for optimal health is at the centre of the wellness vs sickness debate.

Every day, we have to take care of our body
- chose healthy food, real food supplement, exercise, relaxing rest.

Which plants are used for Saccharides?

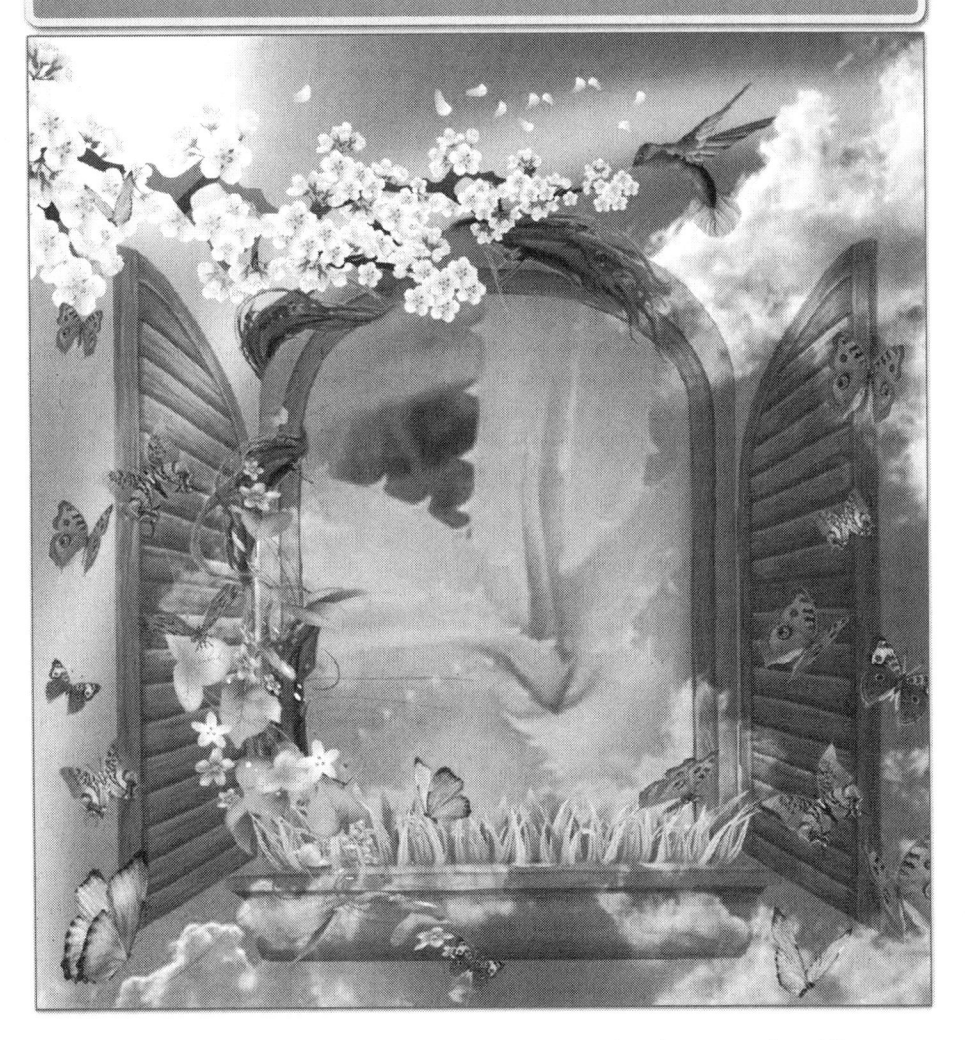

"Let food be your medicine and medicine be your food."

These words are attributed to the ancient Greek physician Hippocrates (460-377 BC), the founding father of natural medicine and the originator of the Hippocratic Oath!

Natural Sources of Saccharides

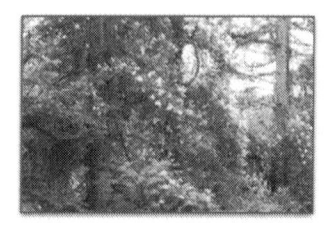

Not surprisingly, many of the sources of Saccharides, especially the essential Saccharides, have been used for centuries as healing medicinal compounds in many cultures around the world.

The primary sources of Saccharides are fungi, saps, gums, and seeds, while the secondary sources are grains, fruit and vegetables.

Glyconutritional mushrooms and fungi

Mushrooms and fungi have been used medicinally in Japan and China for centuries with good results. They contain glucose, galactose and mannose which are known immune system boosters. They have anti-tumour actions, suppress inappropriate immune reactions, and act as modulators of the immune system.

Mushrooms contain a polysaccharide containing beta-glucans, called lentinant, which stimulates the white blood cells to devour invaders and detoxify or clean up the toxins they leave behind. The beta-glucans have been shown to fight cancer and tumour growth thus extending cancer survival time, fight infection in people who have suffered traumatic injuries and protect people from going into shock from severe infections, improve recovery from radiation treatments, and boost wound healing.

Saps and gums

Gum acacia from the African acacia tree contains galactose, rhamnose, arabinose, and glucuronic acid. Gum acacia has been shown to promote healing of irritated gastrointestinal mucosa and respiratory tract tissue, improve beneficial intestinal flora, control colon bifidus fermentation, and lowers triglyceride production, and serum cholesterol.

Gum ghatti from the gum of the Indian sumac contains galactose, arabinose, mannose, xylose, and glucuronic acid. The three essential Saccharides in this gum are important for cell-cell communication and lowering cholesterol. This gum is also beneficial for bifidus fermentation.

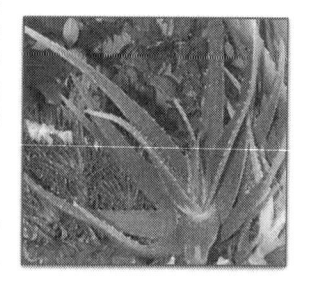

Latrix deciduai or larch tree contains arabinogalactan. Arabinogalactan studies show it has an anti-inflammatory and anti-allergic benefit. It also has been shown to block liver lectins what mediate tumour metastisis; block settling sarcoma L01 tumour ells, and protects intestinal mucosa against disease ad cancer promoting agents. Arabinogalactan also aids recovery from chronic fatigue syndrome.

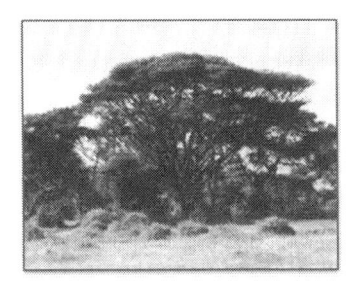

Astragalus gummifer

The Saccharides in the stem and branches of Astragalus gummifer are galactose, arabinose, xylose, fucose, rhamnose, and galcturonic acid. The benefits include action as an antioxidant, diuretic, anti-inflammatory. It inhibits tumour growth, offsets the immune suppression of cancer chemotherapy. Astragalus gummifer also stimulates synthesis of antibodies, delays the natural aging process of blastocysts (fertilised egg cells) by one third, increases the number of stem cells in marrow and lymph and stimulates stem cell development into active immune cells.

Seaweed - Undaria pinnatifida

Undaria pinnatifida, a brown macro seaweed, is one of the richest known sources of in fucose. Fucose influences brain development (fucose is found in human breast milk); acts as an immune modulator; inhibits tumour growth and its spread; and enhances cell-cell communication. High concentrations of fucose are found at the junctions between nerves, in the kidney and testes and in the outer layer of the skin.

Echinacea

Echinacea contains arabinogalactan and galactose and has the benefits gained from the intake of these Saccharides.

Aloe vera

Aloe contains mannose, galactose and arabinose. The leaves are particularly rich in polysaccharides that provide healing and anti-infection properties when used both externally and internally. Aloe acts as an antifungal, antiviral, antibacterial, anti-allergy and antiinflammatory. It also protects the liver from chemical injury.

Taking Saccharides

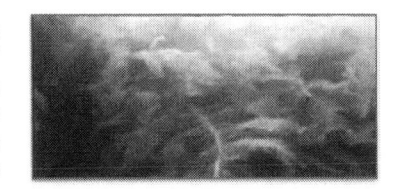

Saccharide supplementation is considered generally safe and non-toxic. Anyone with diabetes should consult their doctor before taking some of the products. Some of the Saccharides products on the market are made from dried fungi or yeasts and people with allergies to these substances need to avoid these products. If you experience fast or irregular breathing, skin rashes, hives, or itching after taking any supplement call your doctor or the company's customer service department. For some of the supplements you need to check with your doctor if you are pregnant or breastfeeding. There are different glyconutritional supplement products on the market and the ingredients and quality standards may vary.

"Glyconutritional formula into a size range compatible with absorption by the body."
One of the emerging fields of scientific research, the human GI tract remains largely an enigma. "There's a lot going on in the GI tract that we are just beginning to understand. It's home to approximately 70 percent of the body's immune system, and previous studies suggest that certain polysaccharides can play an important role in affecting the function of our immune. system. "

Introduction: Why Superfoods?
What Are Superfoods? ... 1

A Note on the Recipes ... 11

The Top 10 Superfoods ... 13

Goji Berries: Fountain of Youth ... 15

Cacao: Raw Chocolate ... 33

Maca: Andes Aphrodisiac ... 67

Bee Products: The Original Superfoods ... 83

   Honey ... 88

   Bee Pollen ... 90

   Royal Jelly ... 93

   Propolis ... 95

Spirulina: Protein Queen ... 107

AFA Blue-Green Algae: Primordial Food
   from Klamath Lake, Oregon ... 123

Marine Phytoplankton: The Basis of All Life ... 145

Aloe Vera: Essene and Egyptian Secret of Immortality .

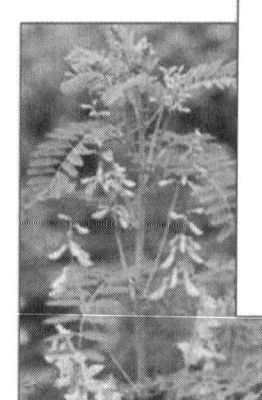

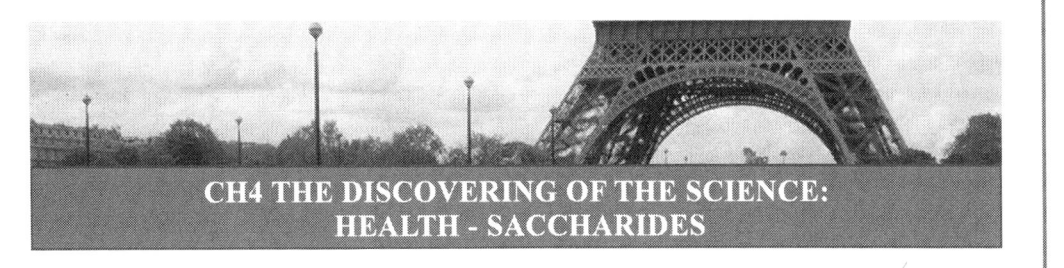

CH4 THE DISCOVERING OF THE SCIENCE: HEALTH - SACCHARIDES

"Almost without exception, whenever two or more living cells interact in a specific way, cell surface carbohydrates will be involved. "- In 1990 the Journal of Biotechnology states.

What is the History of Saccharide Research?

The discovery of the essential Saccharides dates back to the 1980s when Dr Bill McAnalley, a research pharmacologist commenced investigations to determine the active ingredient in Aloe Vera. Several years later he discovered the active ingredient was a carbohydrate with many mannose sugar molecules linked together. But it wasn't as simple as just extracting the mannose from the aloe, the mannose needed to be stabilised as it became inactive quite quickly. A method was developed to stabilise mannose and now over 100 patents protect this process in numerous countries.

The research findings commenced to appear in scientific journals such as Glycobiology Journal and Journal of Biotechnology. This period was followed by several years of scientific validation which led eventually to the knowledge of the importance of the essential Saccharides being mainstreamed.

Why every one needs Saccharides ?

If we are alive and have cells, we need the essential Saccharides ; mannose, galactose, glucose, fucose, xylose, N-acetylglucosamine, N-acetylgalactosamine, and N-acetylneuraminic acid. Whether we are suffering from a medical condition or not, our bodies need Saccharides to function.

According to the scientific research evidence it is clear that if our body is suffering from an auto-immune disorder or degenerative condition it can benefit from Saccharides , notably the essential Saccharides . These Saccharides help our body to exercise its incredible ability to heal, repair, regenerate, regulate and protect itself just by giving it the raw materials it is already pre-programmed to use. The evidence is also clear that by the same processes, the necessary Saccharides are essential to maintaining a healthy body in optimal wellness. If we were getting the essential Saccharides in our diet in sufficient quantities, we would not need supplementation, but unfortunately current agricultural practices, leave our foods with few of the essentials.

We often hear is glycosylated but what dose it mean?

Saccharides are necessary for every cell of your body and when you take Saccharide supplements you are attempting to glycosylate all of the cells in your body.

How fast will it work and which cells will be glycosylated?

Our body is made up of over 600 trillion cells. Cells are constantly being born and dying and cells have different life spans ranging from hours to years.

When we take Saccharide supplements we don't know which cells will be glycosylated or how many. According to Dr Steve Nugent in How to Survive a Toxic Planet it is theoretically possible to take an oral dose of Saccharides, which glycosylate 500,000 cells, as an example, and have 100,000 of those cells continue to live on when 400,000 of them will die. The cells that expired are being replaced by cells, which also need to be glycosylated and you may or may not have sufficient Saccharides available at that moment to get that job done. With this in mind it will, in most cases, take months at a minimum to glycosylate the cells you need for your particular health issue. Our body has the ability to use the Saccharides on what it considers to be the most pressing health issue - and this may be one we aren't aware of eg cancer takes many years to become evident.

What is the relationship between Saccharides and Anti-aging – Saccharides and gerontology?

Our body has a remarkable ability to heal itself, but especially as we grow older the effects of daily stress and lack of proper nutrition reduce our body's ability to maintain good health. We don't have to get sick or grow old faster than we need to. We all live in a hostile environment where staying healthy is a major challenge for everyone especially those of us who have had more time to expose our bodies to toxins and inadequate nutritional intakes.

New discoveries in biochemistry, in particular, in glycobiology, provide us with knowledge on how to slow down the aging process and how to maintain optimum health into our 70s, 80s and beyond. No matter what our age, the addition of Saccharides into our health regime will support our body's incredible ability to heal, repair, regenerate, regulate and protect itself. Science has proven that our bodies use Saccharides to prevent infections and diseases, and slow the aging process.

Many chronic diseases that develop late in life have been found to be influenced by earlier poor eating habits or poor nutritional intake. The earlier a balanced nutrition supplementation program is undertaken the greater the opportunity for prevention of the debilitating multi-diseases of aging. But even in later life when we are suffering the effects of earlier nutrition deficit and the debilitating effects of degenerative disease, the addition of nutritional supplements especially Saccharides, can help to lessen the effects of diseases and improve the quality of life for people who are experiencing disease. This allows older people to maintain their independence for longer. It also can shorten the recovery time from illnesses.

If we take a proactive approach to our wellness as we age, we find that we enter a beneficial recursive cycle. By taking nutritional supplements such as Saccharides that have been shown to improve our body's ability to heal, repair, regenerate, regulate and protect itself, we find we feel better – we have more energy and a greater sense of well being. This leads us to want to be more physically active, which in turn enhances our positive attitude. Combined, these actions and attitudes lead to greatly improved wellness, which makes us feel better and better.

* This is a General Information Book. The statements in this book have not been evaluated by the Food and Drug Administration. *These Saccharide Products are not intended to diagnose, treat, cure or prevent any disease. In any important case with Medical Conditions /diseases, please contact with your doctor.

Joyful heart is a good medicine.

Why do people share Saccharides - new healing science?

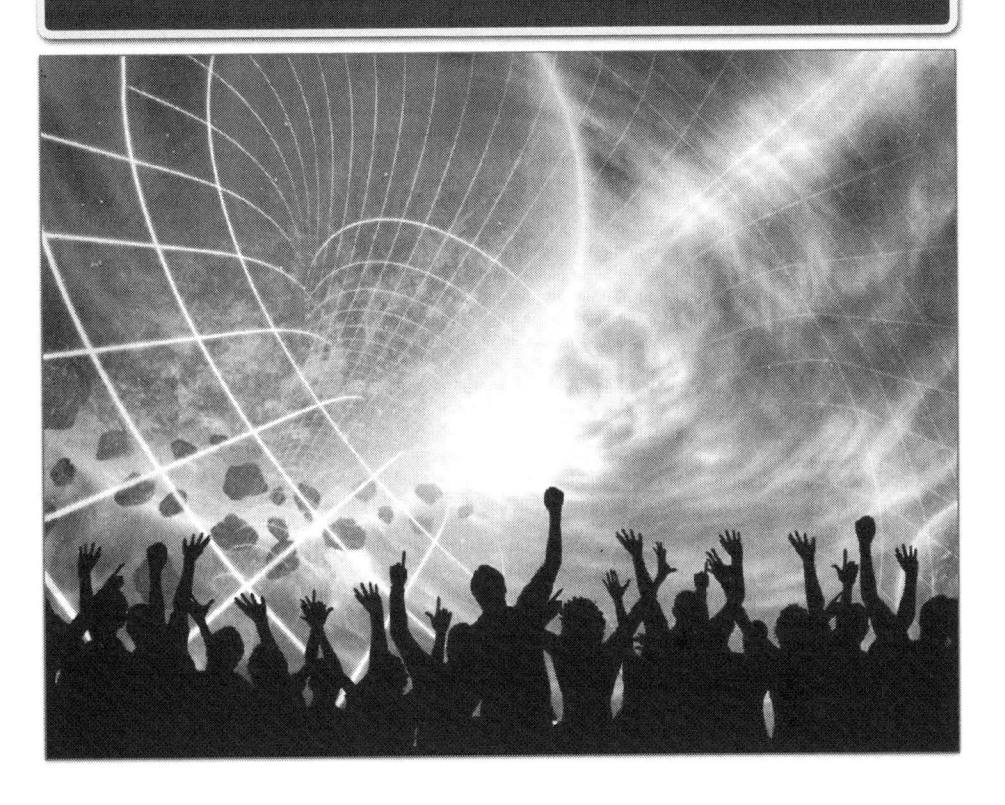

"There are two obstacles to vibrant health and longevity: ignorance and complacency."

~ World Health Organization

Like Vitamins and Mineral, Saccharides are a newly recognized by scientists, as class of nutrients which should ideally be obtained from a good acids and •Monosaccharides. They are well worth looking into by anyone interested in or concerned about their current or future health.

How do scientists react about Saccharides?

There is a LOT of science behind them and thousands of independent scientific studies. Las Vegas Magazine reported the incredible healing story of Greg Letourneau, Executive of the MGM Grand in Las Vegas, whose 10 doctors had given up on him because he was rapidly losing his life with streptococcal toxic-shock syndrome. Then one doctor, Michael Schlachter, MD introduced Saccharides to Letourneau - saving his life. Letourneau beat the odds in Vegas with Saccharides! There are a number of books on the subject including"The Healing Power of 8 Sugars" co-authored by 20 doctors " .

@ Saccharides are not intended to diagnose, treat, cure or prevent any disease, why do people share healing stories ?
Chances are that you know friends and family just like the ones giving their stories here. Loved ones who have tried every medical modality available with less than satisfactory results. The people sharing these stories here have found something new Saccharides. Instead of fighting disease... they are letting nature do the work for them by giving their bodies what the body absolutely needs to function properly. With nutrition and Saccharides in particular. we are not suppressing or manipulating symptoms as with pharmaceuticals. We are not treating conditions as with herbology. We are simply giving the body what it needs to heal itself and rebuild itself anew. These testimonies are shared with you to prove a point. They are not magical, but your body has an extraordinary ability to HEAL and CURE itself when supported by the proper nutrition. Here you will find people who discovered the New Saccharides Technology and to them and their families it "Made a BIG Difference" . We thank them deeply for sharing the good news of new life with new friends in the new science world.

I've been fighting Crohn's as a professional wrestler since 1988. It took me nine years to pin Crohn's. My mission in life is to fight Crohn's. I talk to people all over the U.S. about my fight with Crohn's. In 1988 I was informed that I had Crohn's, no cure. The disease could attack anywhere on the body from the anus to the lips. My doctor told me that my colon was destroyed and it should be removed. Some of the side effects I had were drug- induced diabetes, irregular heartbeat, blood clots, cataracts, and dehydration - which resulted in a 911 call. I developed a hernia. In 1997 my doctor told me the colon had to be removed. It had gotten uglier.

Fortunately, a longtime friend convinced me to try some of these new Saccharides. I was extremely skeptical. He was persistent and I tried them. After three weeks my health improved dramatically. I have my life back and even get in the ring occasionally. In 1998 my doctor told me that I was cured and my colon could be reconnected. This was only after nine months. That

There are four classes as • Vitamins and Mineral •Anino acids •fatty acids and •Saccharides. They make our cells, tissues and organs well in our body. Our best doctor is our immune system: resistant to a particular infection or toxin owing to the presence of specific antibodies or sensitized with blood cells. Saccharides rule supreme in immune system.

Cells
Tissues
Organs
Body

gave me my life back and it is why I'm on this mission to share with others what has so changed my life. The surgeon told me that every place I had growths, fistula and polyps, was a potential malignancy. But I believe that my miracle is not finished yet. ~ Jim ~

Rob Ortmann, MD Immunlogist and Research Scientist
May the Lord our God, through His son Jesus and by the power of the Holy Spirit, open your hearts, mind and spirit to receive this truth and act on it. Father, in the name of Jesus, I proclaim that all these people will have the money to pay for an abundance of Saccharides and that I will be the channel through whom this is accomplished.

Ovarian Carcinoma : I was told by my doctor that I had ovarian carcinoma, stage three to four.

One tumor grew through my colon causing a blockage. The surgeon removed the tumors and repaired the colon. The surgery weakened my colon and it burst a few days later. Soon pelitonitis spread through my abdomen. The doctor later told me they didn't think I'd live another couple months.
1997, I tried the Saccharides. Not only did my tumor growth slow way down, but also my memory and clarity of mind were almost immediately recovered. My strength and stamina began to return. My neuropathy recovered about 70 percent and I did not catch one infection. Although I had another bout with cancer (this time ovarian cancer), I continued with the Saccharides. ~ Crystal ~

Premenopause : About 3 years ago I was experiencing all of the symptoms of Premenopause:

frequent headaches, irritability, sore breasts, bloating and unbelievable "brain fog." I spent most afternoons napping. I didn't even care if I got up to make supper. I decided I needed some help, but I wanted to avoid taking the standard estrogen replacements.
At this time a friend introduced me to the Saccharides. After reading some information, I became excited to find out that they could help my body overcome the pain of arthritis in my knees, shoulders, and hands. My joints hurt every time I walked down stairs or on uneven ground. In just a few days I noticed positive changes. For the first time in ten years I felt an urge to take a

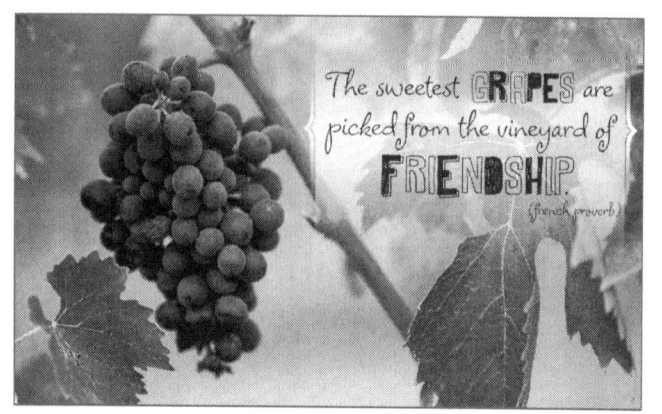

The sweetest GRAPES are picked from the vineyard of FRIENDSHIP.
(french proverb)

walk! The worst of the PMS symptoms, the headaches, bloating and brain fog - disappeared within a month. No more naps, and I wake up each morning feeling refreshed. Also, in four months I lost twenty-five pounds, and have kept them off for nearly three years. My entire family uses the Nutraceuticals. We choose prevention measures as opposed to disease management. ~ Dicksey

Multiple Sclerosis: I was diagnosed with multiple sclerosis in November 1997. I began taking 60 milligrams of Prednisone for double vision. I did not like taking Prednisone as it wiped out my immune system, and made me feel sick and grouchy. When I started to taper off the Prednisone I went to my primary care doctor who suggested I try the Saccharides. At the time I had not done any research on Multiple Sclerosis. I was in complete denial. After Multiple Sclerosis for fifteen years before I was diagnosed. Also, for years I had suffered from severe premenstrual syndrome. After three months on the product, I no longer cry over nothing or act like the Wicked Witch of the West.

Thanks to the Saccharides I can now say the nightmare is over. ~ Diane

Rheumatoid Arthritis/Fibromyalgia : Five years ago I began to swell in different joints. My right arm was constantly swollen from my hand up to my elbow. The pain and stiffness gradually worsened. I literally hurt from the top of my head to the bottom of my feet. After three months of trying every vitamin available, I made an appointment to see a rheumatologist. The diagnosis was fibromyalgia. He gave me a cortisone shot because my left hand was so swollen my wedding band was cutting into my finger. I had four to six weeks reprieve from the pain. In the months that followed I pursued natural remedies.

Eventually I came upon some information on the Saccharides. I decided to try it. I immediately felt an improvement in my energy level. Whenever I slacked off using the strategies, I could feel a setback in my health. I feel significantly better now - and am only taking 2.5 milligrams of Prednisone now. I still have a ways to go - but the last two months I have felt almost normal - a feeling I did not imagine I would ever have again. ~ Sharon ~

Charcot-Marie-Tooth Disease : In 1995 I was diagnosed with Charcot-Marie-Tooth Disease (CMT Type 1A). CMT is a slowly progressive neuropathy causing deterioration of peripheral nerves that control sensory information along with degeneration and muscular atrophy of the lower legs, feet, forearms and hands. Causes problems with balance, muscle cramping, foot-drop walking gait, loss of some normal reflexes, and Scoliosis. The symptoms of CMT are very painful and there is no cure. I could not stand up barefooted and had lost all fat padding. By October 2001 the rate of atrophy in my extremities reached the point that my Podiatrist said there was nothing more he could do for me. My Neurologist confirmed that I had lost all muscular activity from my knees down and the muscles in hands were beginning to atrophy. Soon I would be confined to a wheelchair.

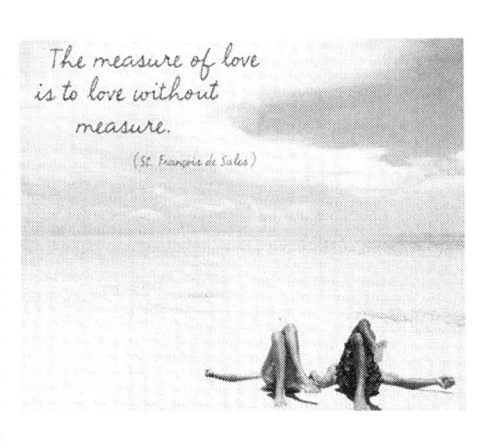

The measure of love is to love without measure.
(St. François de Sales)

In November 2001 I started taking Saccharides. After 2 days a MIRACLE happened, I was able to move my feet and toes! Within 2 weeks my perpetually frozen feet were now feeling warm, I was able to balance and walk without the aid of a walker, and have more energy than ever before! These products have truly changed my life and I am so thankful to have found this wonderful gift. ~ Michele

Depression, Candida Albicans : I believe my problems started to surface and snowball while I was in college. 1996, I hit absolute rock bottom and realized something was wrong with me. I wanted to sleep all the time, I was nasty to people when I was trying so hard to be nice, and I was very depressed. The doctor I worked for prescribed pills and I got very ill. I began to look for a natural route.

My mom heard about the Saccharides and the awesome testimonies of people we knew that had chronic fatigue and Candida problems. After four months before I began to notice signs of change, my energy level started to rise and anxiety attacks were less intense. I am even-tempered and can exercise without becoming totally exhausted, and people began to notice my eyes looked clearer and more alert! Overall, I am still healing but am being patient as my health & well being continue to improve. ~ Cameo

Diabetes : I had lived with diabetes for over thirty-six years and was taking insulin three times a day. I had diabetic related renal disease and eye problems, five coronary bypasses ten years ago, and a heart attack five years ago. My doctors assured me that the complications from the diabetes would only worsen, and a tear in my left rotatator cuff meant that I would never regain full use of my arm. They didn't know why my knee hurt - I'd have to live with it. I was seriously looking for something to make me feel better.

After trying various health foods, I tried the Saccharides. Three months later I noticed that my sugars were going down, pressure was down, and the pain in my knee had lessened. Things just kept getting better. My insulin requirements are down 20 percent. I'm off all blood pressure medicine, and my knee is pain-free. Also, my eyes have improved so much I need a weaker prescription. And, I now have full use of my left arm. Basically, I have a lot more energy and am enjoying life much more. ~ Corrie

Acid Reflux, Arthritis, and Fibroid Tumors.
Within about two weeks of beginning to use some of the Saccharides that a friend shared with me, my stomach problems - acid indigestion and reflux - cleared up. I haven't taken an antacid since. And I can eat foods that I wasn't able to eat before. The arthritis in my hands also cleared up. But the most remarkable thing that happened is within four months of making some changes, my fibroid tumors were gone! (My gynecologist verified this.) Because I was so impacted by my health recovery experience, I gave up my twenty-six-year career as a real estate appraiser and writer of continuing education materials for appraisers in order to help people in the way I was helped. ~ Peggy

Metastatic Melanoma : "You have, maximum, six months to live," said my oncologist eight years ago. Having seen three other patients of his die within five months of metastatic melanoma, I knew he was telling the truth. So I said, "No" to his proposed chemo treatments. We prayed to the Lord for guidance and started looking for answers.
After weeks of natural therapy and new orientation in Mexico, we began a whole new life based on the principles of WELLNESS. I've done well. I am now the Florida State Champion in the 5K-race walk among men aged seventy to seventy-four. But in spite of all the grace of God and victory of these years, my intense search for the best therapy was getting confusing.

Gulf War Syndrome: I am a Gulf War veteran and I have had many of the symptoms of Gulf War syndrome. Some of those ailments include: headaches, severe fatigue, aching joints, sore muscles, memory loss, abdominal pain, huge bleeding boils, severe nausea, and severe mood swings. Before I started the nutraceuticals, I was not very happy with life. I was not suicidal, but I was not much fun to be around. I did not feel like doing anything.
After I started the Saccharides a friend shared with me, I started feeling like a normal person again. I started having more fun with my family and actually wanted to go out and do things. I always feel the drive and energy to do whatever I want to do. ~ Ettor

"I really believe that Saccharides are something that will become mandatory for overall health, and the reason I have come to these conclusions is because I have spent the past several months doing what I call research on the research. And when I would do searches on Saccharides, and especially a lot of different disease processes, I was floored by the number of quality studies that are out there that have shown such benefit and promise in a myriad of diseases ranging from diabetes to arthritis." Arthritis several years ago my knee was injured playing basketball. An orthopedic surgeon told me I had the knee of an eighty-year-old. I was thirty-eight at the time. I was too young for knee replacement surgery, so I just had to live with the pain. My wife had been in an automobile accident, so she too was facing many physical problems.

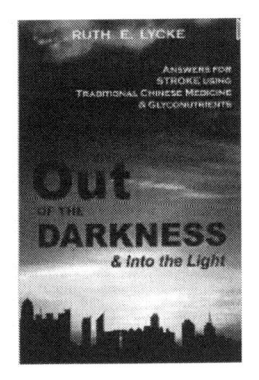

A close friend of ours suggested the Saccharides for both of us. After only two weeks the pain in my knee was gone- even after standing on it all day. My wife experienced tremendous changes in hormonal areas, including no premenstrual symptoms and regular cycles for the first time in thirty years! Our energy levels and overall health have improved noticeably. ~ Jerry

Out of the Darkness and into the Light: Answers for Stroke Using Traditional Chinese Medicine & Saccharides Ruth E. Lycke (Author) November 11, 2005

Ruth suffered a brain stem bleed and subsequent stroke in November of 2001. Expected to die within the first 24 hours she battled back and lived. Overcoming horrific odds she progressed slowly through the recovery process. As a faithful patient Ruth followed all of her physicians recommendations. 2 1/2 years later she had regained far more than her doctors thought possible. Still 100% disabled she was encouraged by her physicians to accept her condition and be content

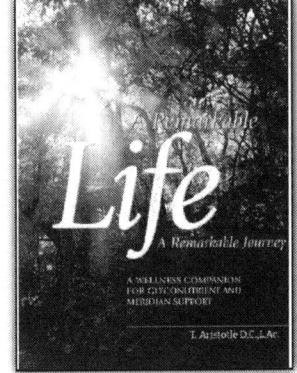

Fibromyalgia and Manic Depression : Over eighteen years ago I was diagnosed with fibromyalgia and manic depression. I spent two weeks at General Hospital for the depression. Every day when I awoke I wished I were dead. I prayed to God to help me get through the day. I also spent three months in therapy. I thought I was getting better, but then the pain became worse than ever. I was put on a lot of medications like Prozac, Amitripaline, and many others. It gave me numerous bad side effects.

My sister told me about one of the five strategies to vibrant health and longevity. My depression got so bad I wouldn't get out of bed for fear I would do something bad to myself. I finally got desperate and called my sister I asked her about some of the Saccharides for health she had told me about. Within three days of using Saccharides, the fog lifted and I was no longer . I now have my life back. My doctor can't believe I'm no longer depressed. I don't see counselors or psychiatrists anymore. My husband, who now follows some of the same strategies I do, no longer has angina attacks. I've met so many wonderful people in this business of sharing the keys to health. I am so thankful to have my life back - and I love helping other people feel the same. ~ Jackie

We express gratitude to them for sharing the good news of new life stories with new friends in the new science world.

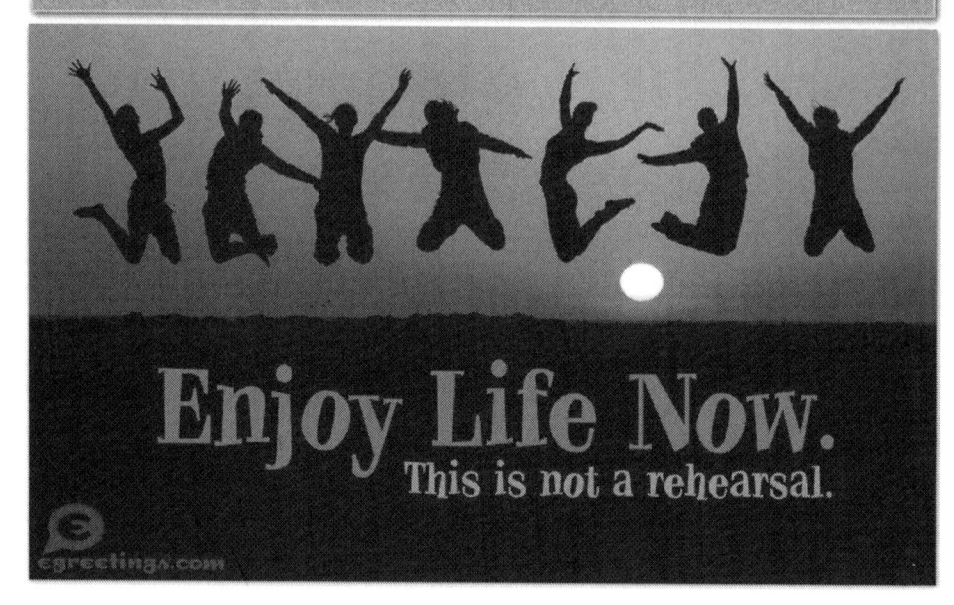

Enjoy Life Now.
This is not a rehearsal.

with what little she had regained. Faced with seemingly insurmountable odds Ruth refused to be content was determined to begin a quest to regain all that she had lost. It took years after the stroke for her to discover the answers that would end her suffering with "disabilities" and restore the person she once was. Follow Ruth as she journeys out of the darkness of the stroke. Experience the tears and joys, frustration and hope, as she uncovers answers in ancient mysteries in a far away land. Join her on the quest that finally brought her into the light. NEVER SAY NEVER!

Life :   T. Aristotle is a Doctor of Chiropractic and serves on the faculty of The International Academy of Medical Acupuncture. This academy is an institute of higher learning dedicated to teaching physicians of all disciplines the ancient principles of acupuncture as well as the technologically advanced Contemporary Chinese Medicine (CCM) techniques & procedures . New and Updated products are included for personalized Saccharides support. Over 300 health conditions with current Saccharides and acupupressure point recommendations;

Over 300 meridian diagrams with point location . Clinical pressure points for each condition . Meridian Therapy . Tips for hospital settings.

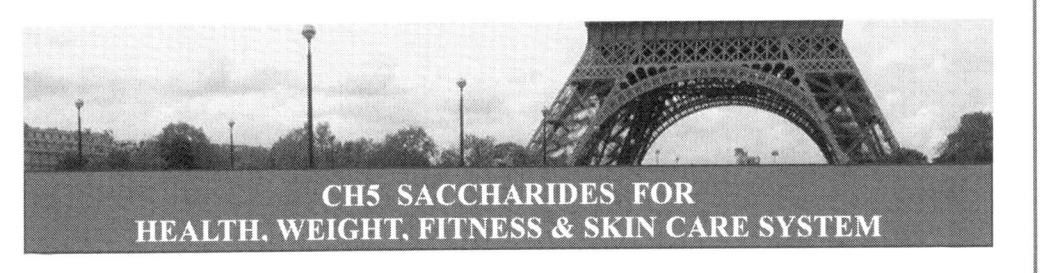

CH5 SACCHARIDES FOR HEALTH, WEIGHT, FITNESS & SKIN CARE SYSTEM

With our Real Food Technology Solution, we prefer to get our vitamins, minerals, phytonutrients and other plant-sourced ingredients from thinks that are genuinely food and put them in a form that's easy for people to take every day.

Where can we get more information about SACCHARIDES PRODUCTS?
If you search around Internet, you will get more details on the discovery, invention and science research about Saccharides.

What Are Antioxidants?
Antioxidants are substances that, even in relatively low concentrations, significantly inhibit the rate of oxidation caused by FROs. Antioxidants can be classified into groups based on how they work and where they are found. For convenience, five major classes of antioxidants have been delineated: natural enzyme antioxidants, natural preventative antioxidants, scavenging antioxidants, dietary antioxidants, and pharmacological antioxidants.1,5

Natural enzyme antioxidants are found in the intracellular environment and include superoxide dismutase (SOD), catalase, and glutathione peroxidase. Catalase is found inside the heme molecule. Glutathione peroxidase contains selenium and helps prevent formation of the highly destructive hydroxyl radical. It regenerates vitamin C, which in turn regenerates vitamin E. It requires nicotinamide-adenine dinucleotide phosphate (NADPH) and is produced from the pentose phosphate pathway.1

References 1. Maxwell SRJ. Prospect for the use of antioxidant therapies. Drugs 1995;49(3):345-361

Why the phytosterols or phytohormones are important for human hormone?

One of the most important groups of phytochemicals are the phytosterols or phytohormones as they are sometimes known. These are plant based sterols that act as precursors to human sterols. They act to modulate the human endocrine system. One of the most important human sterols is Dehydroepiandrosterone (DHEA). This hormone is produced in our adrenal glands and serves a variety of functions. It is often called the 'mother' hormone as it has the ability to convert itself into other hormones such as oestrogen, testosterone, progesterone, and corticosterone, on demand. Thus it is a precursor to all other hormones and active metabolites. Precursors are substances the body uses to produce other substances.

Scientific research reveals that adequate DHEA in the body can slow the aging process, and prevent, improve, and even often reverse conditions such as cancer, heart disease, memory loss, obesity, and osteoporosis. DHEA blood levels peak between ages 20 to 25 years and then decline with age in both men and women. DHEA is the precursor of stress hormones such as cortisol and adrenaline. That is, our body makes cortisol and adrenaline from DHEA. When our body makes these hormones, DHEA levels decline. Dioscorea, found in the Mexican yam, contains a biochemical storehouse of valuable phytochemicals for use as hormone precursors. The molecular structure is almost identical to the body's natural hormone precursors.

Where are Saccharides used for?

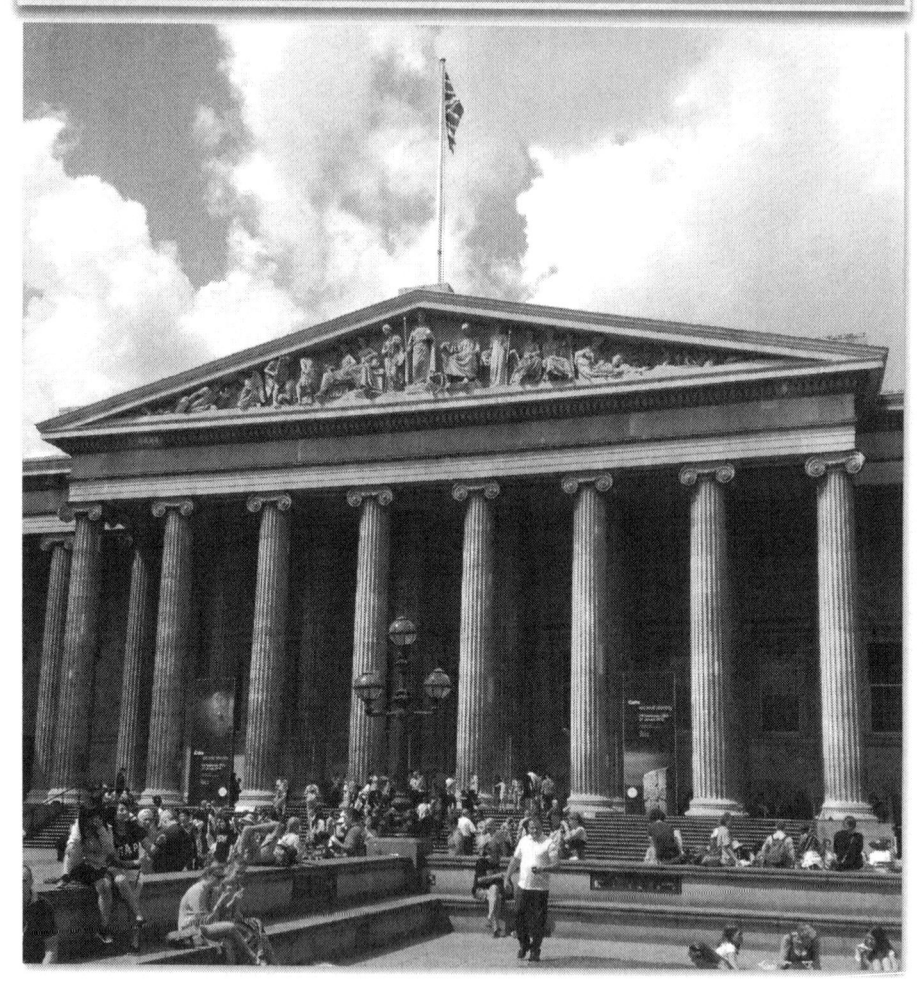

Saccharides is the wellness solution

for the 21st century.

31

Do the foods we eat affect the way we feel?
Absolutely! Anyone who has missed a meal appreciates the surge of energy and the feeling of well-being that a good meal provides.

But what about the effects of foods or dietary supplements on how we feel in a broader sense?
Sometimes, response to dietary changes may be obvious and rapid, such as improved energy levels and a renewed sense of well-being. However, long-term, good health depends on a body built with healthy cells. The question then becomes, "How long will it take before my dietary changes build new, perhaps healthier cells?"

For fundamentals of Human Cells, how often are new cells made?
That depends on the type of cell. Our bodies are composed of about 200 different cell types. Only a few are never replaced; these "immortal" cells include auditory hair cells, heart muscle cells, and nerve cells.

What about the rest of the cell types?
The table below provides lifespan information for some of the remaining 197 types.*1,2. of supplementation. At six months, however, significant improvements in all measures were found, despite heavier training activity (which can depress RBC status). *3 Studies examining the effects of nutrient deprivation and repletion are limited. The few studies that have been performed often reveal the large variability of response between individuals and emphasize the delay before these nutrients take effect.

What does all this Studies mean?
While some cells are rapidly replaced, many others survive for months – or even years! So it can take months or longer before our changed dietary habits can profoundly affect our cells. Some people experience a rapid response to dietary changes. For many, however, dietary improvements must be sustained for at least a few months before cellular function can be expected to improve.

Let's consider vitamin C, How long will it take before my dietary changes build new, perhaps healthier cells?
Two studies on vitamin C reported that individual responses to vitamin C deprivation (and supplementation) were highly variable. 1.2.The first sign of vitamin C depletion took roughly one month to appear; by the fourth month of deprivation, 1/3 of the participants had almost completely depleted their bodily reserves, but the other 2/3 continued to have acceptable amounts. Following supplementation a return to normal plasma levels often took well over a month, and in some cases 100 days was required.

See LIFESPAN OF SOME CELLS OF THE HUMAN BODY, how often are new cells made?

LIFESPAN OF SOME CELLS OF THE HUMAN BODY	
CELL TYPE	**LIFESPAN**
Granulocytes: eosinophils, basophils, neutrophils	10 hours - 3 days
Stomach lining cells	2 days
Colon cells	3-4 days
Epithelia of small intestine	1 week or less
Platelets	10 days
Skin epidermal cells	2-4 weeks
Lymphocytes	2 months – more than a year (highly variable)
Red blood cells	4 months
Macrophages	Months-years
Endothelial cells	Months-years
Bone cells	25-30 years

What does all this Clinical Studies mean?
Few studies have examined cellular response to nutritional change. In one study of 16 distance runners consuming nutritional supplements designed to improve red blood cell (RBC) status, no improvement was noted after one month.

What are the difference between Saccharides and eating sugar like candy?
While Saccharides are sometimes referred to as "sugars" or "nature's sugars", they are different from the sugar (sucrose) in unhealthy foods like sugary soft drinks or candy. Most people eat entirely too much sucrose, a disaccharide that raises blood glucose and insulin levels and is one of many culprits contributing to our current obesity epidemic. The Saccharides sugars are healthy, fiber-rich complex plant saccharides that do not affect blood glucose levels.

Do you know A Little History on Aloe Vera?
Aloe Vera - the medicinal values of this wonderful herb have been known for centuries. A 3500 year old document (Papyrus Ebers) at the Leipzig University describes Aloe and it's values as a medicine.

The Chinese were recorded to have used Aloe between 772 and 842 on eczematous rashes and again between 960 and 1276 it was used for the treatment of eczema.

Medicinal applications were made by Dioscorides 2000 years ago for healing wounds, insomnia, ulcers, hemorrhoids, itching, skin care, blemishes, mouth and gum diseases and the loss of hair.
The use of Aloe was noted by W. Turner in 1568 and by J.R. Coxe in 1818 for the use of healing wounds. These are described in the publications of Herbal and The Dispensatory of the United States of America respectively.

Jamaicans are said to relieve headaches with Aloe. Spanish missionaries frequently carried it with them upon visiting the sick. Seminole Indians applied Aloe to incisions after surgery.

Mexican Indians used it for all sorts of stomach and intestinal disorders, longevity, bladder and kidney infections and also for prostatitis. The prevention of scars from wounds and the improvement of the scalp and growth of hair have been the reason for the use of Aloe in Java.

Survivors of the A-Bomb blast in Japan tell of the use of Aloe to treat radiation burns. This in truth prompted the Los Alamos Scientific Laboratory for the United States Atomic Energy Commission to test Aloe Vera on radiation burns. The results showed complete healing in two months as compared to the untreated area which was still not completely healed after four months.

What is Aloe Vera?

The Aloe Vera plant is a succulent perennial and a species of plant belonging to the Lily family which is part of a larger family of plants known as "Xeroids". Of the known medicinal Aloes, Aloe Barbadensis Miller has the Greatest medicinal activity and is the only Aloe bearing the botanical name Aloe Vera, Vera meaning true in Latin, Thus "True Aloe" or "Aloe Vera".

What are the Substances Found in Aloe Vera?
According to Stanford University of California and the University of Tennessee researchers and other scientists, substances reported to occur in Aloe Vera gel include polysaccharides containing glucose, mannose, tannins, steroids, organic acids, antibiotic principles, glucuronic acid, enzymes, (oxidase, catalase, and amylase), trace sugar, calcium oxalate, a protein containing 18 amino acids, "wound healing hormones", biogenic stimulators, sapoin, vitamins, and mineral: chloride, sulfate, iron, calcium copper, sodium, potassium, manganese, magnesium, silicon, and phosphatide esters.

What are the ingredients found in Aloe Vera juice and gel?

The following ingredients found in our Aloe Vera juice and gel are: Potassium Sorbate is used as a preservative to counteract bacteria. Ascorbic Acid is an anti-oxidant, also known as Vitamin C. Citric Acid is used as a preservative. The gel has minute amount of Xanthan Gum in order to provide that wonderful coating action.

The rate of increase in incidence of autoimmune and degenerative diseases is alarming, especially when we look at the dramatic rate of increase of these diseases in our children. Allopathic medicine has failed to halt this increase, and can only prescribe drugs with some very serious, and in some cases, life threatening side effects. In fact when we look at cause of death, properly prescribed, properly administered (in hospital) pharmaceutical agents, ranks as No. 4 behind strokes, cancer and heart disease.

Modern medicine or allopathic medicine is now facing the need for a total paradigm shift in its thinking – as deep a shift as the one that occurred when bacteria were first shown to be the agents of infectious diseases, and not 'bad air'. Years of treating sickness and symptoms rather than promoting wellness and finding causes have led to an urgent need for all of us to take greater responsibility for our health.

There is scientific evidence that our health problems are related to a combination of nutritional deficiency and environmental toxicity. There is also a growing appreciation of the body's natural physiological capabilities to support health and wellness. This movement towards wellness began slowly but is now rapidly gaining momentum as the affluent Baby Boomer generation leads the way with a commitment to retaining their wellness. Their commitment is to be proactive and prevent ill health and degenerative and autoimmune diseases rather than waiting until their onset and then treating the symptoms. Wellness is different to health. 'Health' is what we see or feel. We may feel and look healthy but could be harbouring cancer or heart disease. Often the first symptom of heart disease is a heart attack, but the disease has often been developing for many years. The wellness revolution is based on giving the body what it needs to support optimal health (both seen and unseen) and quality of life.

Toxins, Free Radicals and Anti-oxidants.

We all live in a toxic environment. No matter where we live or how careful we are, we can't avoid environmental toxins. They are in the air we breathe, the food we eat and the water we drink all over the planet. What is particularly worrying is the high levels of pesticides in our homes, considerably higher to levels we are exposed to outdoors.

Free radicals are produced when our cells create energy and when we are exposed to pollutants or toxins such as cigarette smoke, alcohol or pesticides. If allowed to go unquenched, free radicals can cause damage to the body's cells. The cells that line the arteries, the fat cells in the blood, the immune cells and so on can all be affected by free radicals. And because of this, free radical damage (or oxidation) has been linked to the formation of every degenerative disease known including cancer, cardiovascular disease, cataracts and the ageing process itself.

Free radicals are unstable chemicals formed in the body during normal metabolism or exposure to environmental toxins such as air, food and water pollution. Free radicals help our bodies to generate energy and fight infections, but when we have too many free radicals they attack healthy cells causing them to age prematurely. The action of rust is probably the best analogy of how excess free radicals work in our body.

We are being constantly exposed to increasing amounts of free radicals due to increasing environmental toxins in our living and working environment. At the same time our intake of protective cell pigments is decreasing. Free radicals are known to cause or exacerbate most (and especially chronic) diseases such as cancer, heart disease, arthritis, diabetes, macular degeneration and cataracts.

Free radical damage mutates the body's future DNA and RNA cell blueprint message by pairing with electrons in the DNA chains, ultimately leading to cellular electronic imbalance. Inevitable blurring of the DNA and RNA blueprint will occur as mutated cells replicate this is aging. In other cases, excess free radical damage can cause DNA messages to accelerate the cell division process into a state of panic whereby DNA are unable to withstand the rate of degeneration - this is cancer.

Why do Children need Saccharides?

The incidence of disease and medical conditions in children is increasing at an alarming rate. In the United States alone there are 59 million children that are considered to have some disability. The leading cause of death of children aged 1-14 years is cancer.

Asthma is reported as the leading cause of chronic illness among children. The Agency for Healthcare Research and Quality reports that, Asthma-related deaths and illnesses have increased in recent years among young people with asthma, who miss school three times as often as other youngsters. The incidence of Attention Deficit Disorder (ADD) and Attention Deficit Deficit

Hyperactivity Disorder (ADHD) has reached almost epidemic proportions, and one half of children diagnosed with ADD or ADHD have been identified as having a learning disability.

There is growing research evidence that ADD/ADHD and other learning disorders are a result of lack of communication within the brain. The vital Saccharides are what is missing to enable its cells to communicate properly. Also since the brain controls the entire body, if it has limited communication then other things start to go wrong.

What was once called; Adult Onset Diabetes (Type II) is no longer called that because an alarming and increasing number of children have been diagnosed with this degenerative disease.

The Centre for Disease Control and Prevention reports that infectious diseases amongst children are on the increase, partly as a result of the over-use of antibiotics. Healthy immune systems would alleviate the need for antibiotics in many instances.

An article in the Journal of Nutritional and Environmental Medicine (1996:6), titled Effective Nutritional Medicine: The application of nutrition to major health problems, states that there is a significant body of convincing, scientific research evidence which clearly shows that nutritional, environmental and lifestyle related factors contribute to present day diseases to a great extent. This cannot be ignored.

Today's diets for the majority of our children have many shortcomings, in many cases diets are grossly inadequate to meet their nutritional needs. Because of the decline in nutritional levels in our food, even when children eat fruit and vegetables it is almost impossible for them to meet their daily nutritional needs.

What are the benefits of glyconutritional supplementation in children?

The benefits of glyconutritional supplementation in children:

- Significantly enhanced brain functioning with an ability to focus longer, learn and retain information easier, and reductions in behaviour challenges.
- Significantly increased academic performance by reversing genetic disorders, decreased incidence of infections, decreased chronic and degenerative health problems.
- Significantly increased athletic/sport performance and endurance, with shorter recovery times, fewer sports injuries.
- Reduced absentecism from school and extra-curricular activities due to illness or injury.
- Reduced healthcare costs for the whole family - fewer trips to the general practitioner and fewer pharmaceutical drugs.

The bottom line is Saccharides supplementation allows the body to exercise its incredible ability to heal, repair, regenerate, regulate and protect itself just by giving it the raw materials it is already pre-programmed to use.

Fitness and Health

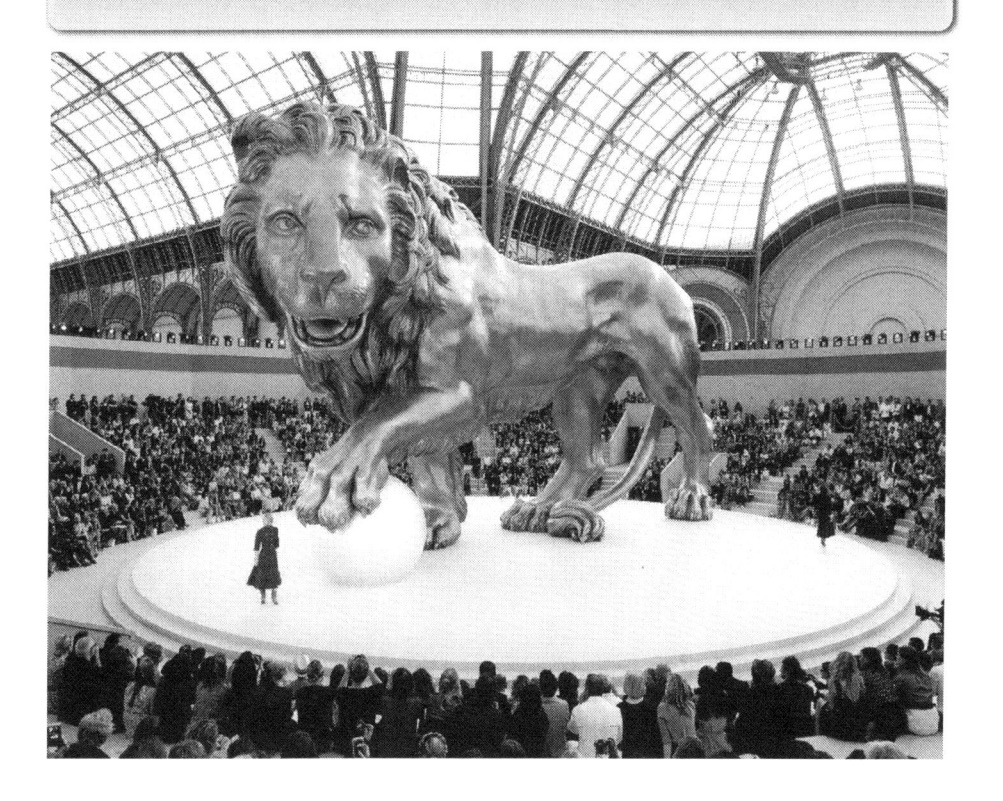

Look younger, feel younger, be young。
#1 New York Times bestseller Bob Greene

> **Achieve the healthy, fit body you want** *
>
> Get fit and lose the weight you want with Real Food Technology® solutions — our method of creating powerful products using the most natural ingredients available. Clinically tested and proven to work, advanced weight and fitness products are natural and endurance-formulated with powerful, food-sourced nutrients to help you go the extra mile, and look amazing while doing it.

Inactivity and Weight Gain—Which Comes First?

Presentations on BBC News, researchers have challenged the assumption that weight gain, particularly in children, is caused by a lack of exercise. The investigators followed a group of more than 200 children for 11 years, regularly monitoring body fat and exercise. Their findings suggest that rather than weight gain being caused by a lack of exercise, it is somewhat opposite—excess weight gain causes a decrease in activity. The researchers published their findings in a journal1 and concluded that to effectively find solutions to excessive weight gain, we need to focus more on food consumption than on exercise.

Why do Athletes use Saccharides?

Nutrition is paramount for athletes seeking to achieve maximal performance and rapid post-exercise recovery. For elite athletes dietary factors can often translate into those milliseconds that separate winning from losing. Glyconutrition can support athletes in increasing performance, reducing pain, and reducing recovery time.

Optimised cellular function through Saccharides supplementation results in enhanced performance. Roy Kurban, a karate black belt and Black Belt Magazine's previous Man of the Year had tried many new nutritional supplements before he started taking Saccharides in 1996. He found that Saccharides worked where others didn't.

A study involving NFL athletes found that those taking Saccharides experienced less pain, had an improved range of motion in their joints and experienced an overall improvement in their quality of life.

One of the major drawbacks of the intensive training regimes undertaken by elite athletes is the diminished immune system function, resulting in increased risk of infection, prolonged recovery time and decreased tissue repair mechanisms. Saccharides boost immune system functioning and support the natural functions of our body to heal, repair, regenerate, regulate and protect itself.; Antioxidants can help protect your cells from free radicals which are released during exercise.

It's well known that excessive exercise diminishes immune-system function. This increases the risk of infection, prolongs recovery time and decreases tissue-repair mechanisms. Saccharides have been shown to enhance immune function. Both the

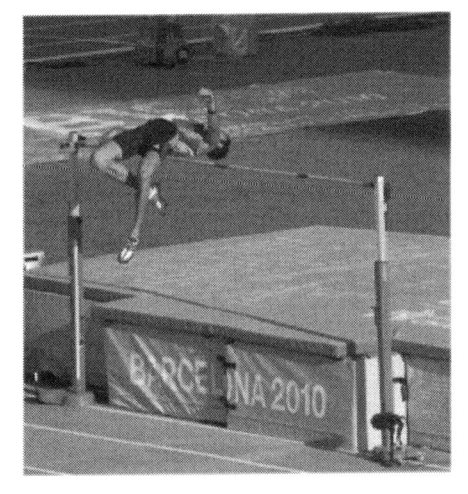

U.S. and Canadian Olympic teams officially endorse Saccharide products for their athletes.

Glycoproteins make up more than 85% of the molecules in our cells. If glycosylation is not adequate, due to deficiency in Saccharides, then crucial cells and their components – such as enzymes, antibodies, collagen, muscle fibres, hormones – are not created in sufficient quantities and as a result health and performance can be dramatically reduced.

Saccharides are non-toxic at even high amounts, and there is no possibility of long-term damage or drug interactions.

This is not too surprising when you consider the calorie equivalency of food and exercise. One pound of fat is equivalent to approximately 3,500 calories. In other words, an excess intake of 3,500 calories will add one pound of fat to the body. Looking at calorie tables for some diets, particularly those full of fast foods, 3,500 calories in one sitting is not beyond the reach of some people. To exercise off 3,500 calories, you would have to run a marathon, over 26 miles, something quite beyond the reach of the vast majority of people.

The bottom line is, while exercise has wide health benefits, both physical and psychological, and those benefits must not be downplayed, the main focus for dealing with the global weight problem should be nutrition. Nutrition plus exercise would be optimal.

How to overcome the weight loss hurdles that are unique to women?
(7 Weight Loss Challenges and Tips for Women sharecare.com)

Men and women were created equal, but they are different. Especially when it comes to weight loss. Women face some unique challenges in getting the bathroom scale to budge. And these challenges are both medical and emotional in nature. So whether you're trying to lose 5 pounds or 50, it's important to understand your weight loss challenges. That way, you'll be armed with weight loss tips (specifically for women) and strategies that can help you break through those obstacles and making slimming down easier.

Obstacle #1: Do you feel stressed?

Almost everyone feels stress at some point in the day. But research shows that women are more prone to feeling stress as they juggle the demands of their work commitments, their family lives, and their social ties. And not only that, but women are also more likely than men to feel guilt when work interrupts their home lives. All of that pressure adds up, sending stress-hormone levels soaring.

The kicker in all of this? Research shows that high levels of a stress hormone called cortisol increases appetite. Uh-oh. And cortisol makes people crave foods high in fat and sugar. Double uh-oh.

The solution: To help keep stress from sabotaging your waistline, one of the best weight loss tips for women is to spend at least a few minutes every day practicing a simple stress reduction strategy. Like one of these:

Walk for 10 minutes. (And walk outside if you can.)

Breathe deeply 10 times. (Learn how to use breathing to jumpstart weight loss.)

Tense and then relax each muscle group. (Start at your toes and move up.)

Find a quiet place to meditate for 10 minutes. (Here's a quick guide to meditating.)

Obstacle #2: Are you getting enough sleep?

Most people don't get enough sleep. But women have more sleep struggles than men do. In fact, about 70% of women get fewer than 8 hours of sleep per night. Women have more trouble falling and staying asleep, and they also suffer from more daytime sleepiness compared with men. Some of the top factors in women's sleep troubles include work and family stress, health problems, and uncomfortable beds.

All of which can add up to stubborn pounds, because a lack of sleep throws appetite hormones off and stimulates overeating.

The solution: Sleep in. Go to bed early. Makeover your bedroom until it resembles a veritable sleep-fantasy suite. Do whatever you need to do to get the recommended 7 to 8 hours a night. Especially if you're trying to lose weight. (Try these tips to fall asleep naturally.)

Obstacle #3: Feeling sluggish?

A sluggish thyroid -- also know as an underactive thyroid gland or hypothyroidism -- is much more likely to develop in women than in men, especially after menopause. And that spells trouble for waistlines. Here's why: In addition to fatigue and sluggishness, an underactive thyroid can also cause weight gain.

The solution: If you have unexplained fatigue and weight gain, have your thyroid levels checked. An autoimmune condition called Hashimoto's disease is a frequent cause of hypothyroidism, and it's more common in women than in men. Another underlying cause of hypothyroidism in women: pregnancy. (Is your thyroid going haywire? Look for these signs.)

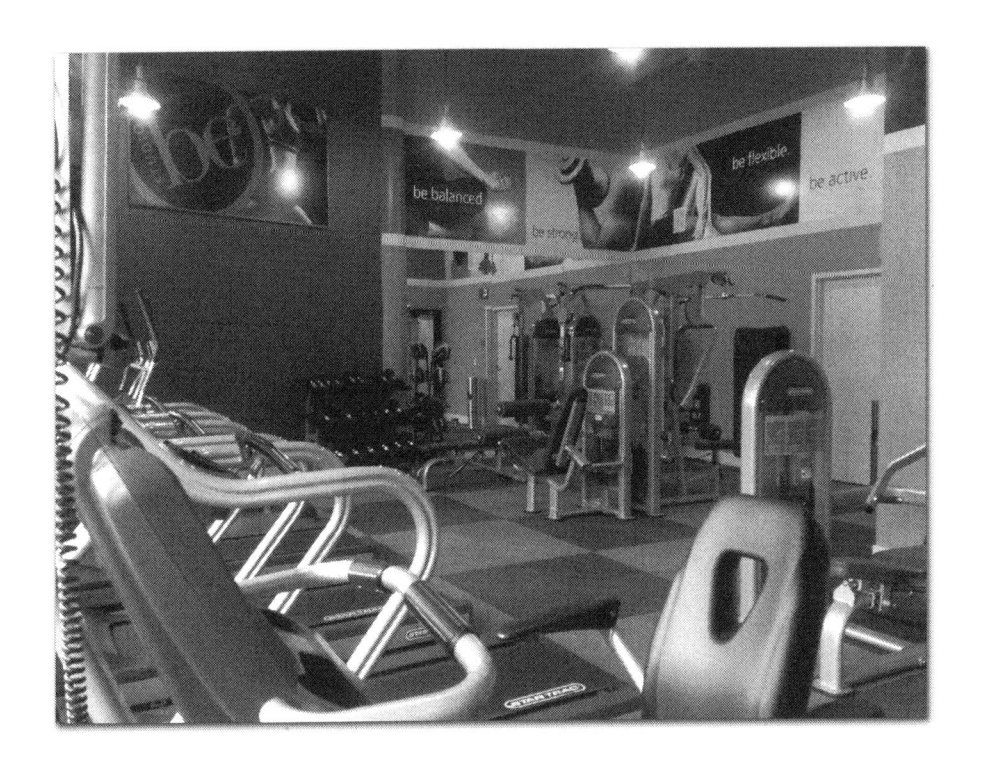

Obstacle #4: How much muscle do you have?

Blame this one on Mother Nature. Women's bodies are built differently than men's -- women have more fat and less muscle. And less lean body mass means they have lower resting metabolic rates compared with men. Women burn fewer calories on a baseline level. And that smaller body size means women burn fewer calories with the same amount of exercise. And their bodies have evolved to hold on to fat stores better, in order to produce and nourish healthy babies.

The solution: Avoid super-low-calorie diets that'll put you into starvation mode and make it harder for your body to burn calories and lose weight. Eat small meals throughout the day so your metabolism stays fired up. Also, focus more of your workout on strength training -- to help you keep the muscle you have. (Watch this video to find out how adding 5 pounds of muscle through strength training can translate into 26 pounds lost.)

Obstacle #5: Feeling hormonal?

As women age, estrogen levels drop and metabolism slows down. And, as a result, women lose muscle and gain fat, especially around the abdomen.

The solution: Amp up your activity. Research shows that as women reach the age of menopause, they tend to exercise less. Make it a priority to walk at least 30 minutes a day most days of the week, rain or shine, year in and year out.

Obstacle #6: Got a craving for cookies?

Studies suggest that women cave into food cravings more easily than men do. Women are also more likely to eat when they are sad or depressed and, in those moments, tend to reach for comfort foods that are high in fat and sugar. It's a recipe for disaster when it comes to trying to lose weight.

The solution: Relying on sheer willpower to curb cravings may not be the way to go. Instead, research suggests you might be better off using a practice called mindfulness meditation -- where you actually spend time acknowledging the craving. By recognizing, experiencing, and feeling the craving, you may be more likely to resist it than if you'd tried to suppress or ignore it. (Learn more about how to use mindfulness meditation to resist cravings better.)

Obstacle #7: Feeling bad about yourself?

Those pretty magazines with the skinny models? Get them out of your house. Those TV shows with the preternaturally preserved faces? Turn them off. Those success stories about women who lost 20 pounds in 1 month? Ignore them. Media images of stick-thin women and unrealistic weight loss goals cause many women to become frustrated and give up their own diet and exercise plans when their results don't match up.

The solution: Be kind to yourself, and don't beat yourself up if you have an occasional treat. Give yourself time to see results. If it took 3 years to put those extra pounds on, it's not unreasonable to give yourself 3 years to get them all off. And if you fall off the wagon, don't throw in the towel. Slips are bound to happen occasionally. Feeling guilty about it is only going to make losing weight harder.

What is the plan?

We chose an all-natural protein blend that in a clinical study targeted fat loss while sparing lean muscle, when combined with a reduced-calorie diet plan and proper exercise.

What ingredients are in the all-natural protein blend powder?

This kind of powder is a specially formulated whey protein blend that includes an advanced protein peptide technology, which helps the body burn fat while maintaining lean muscle.*

Too busy to meet your nutritional needs?

Get the low-glycemic meal replacement drink that gives you nutrients you need without the calories you don't. The real food meal replacement drink mix is a tasty, nutritionally balanced drink for people with busy lifestyles like you. Get the equivalent of a full meal in seconds!Satisfy your hunger while cutting calories. Delicious, low-glycemic the real food meal replacement drink mix comes in rich chocolate and French vanilla flavors and delivers:

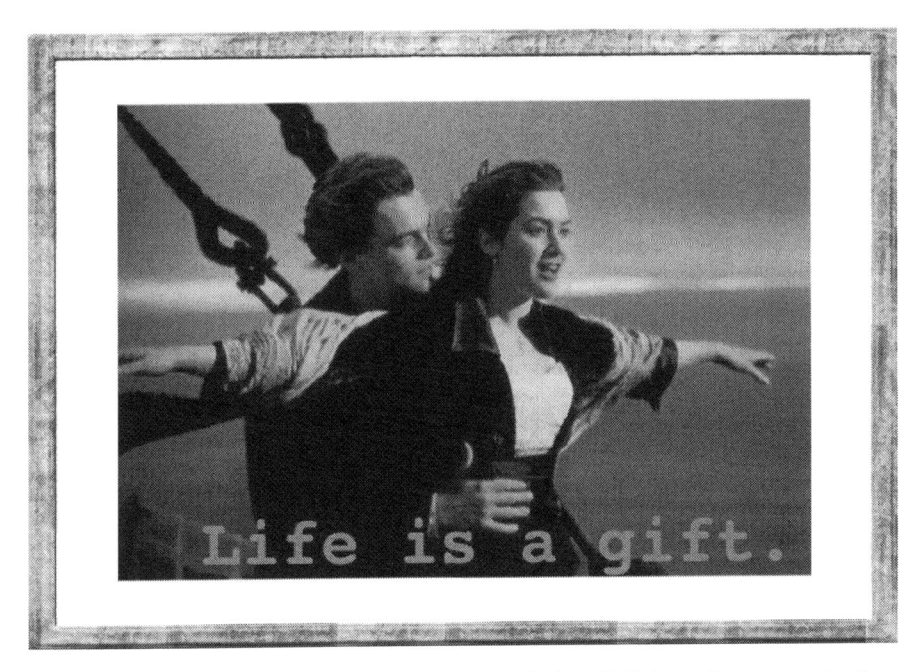

The nutrients your body needs to feel full and satisfied. The essential fatty acids you need to feel your best

Why do we need to do Exercise every day?
There is overwhelming evidence that people who lead active lifestyles are less likely to die early, or to experience major illnesses such as heart disease, diabetes and colon cancer. The evidence shows that regular exercise can:

increase levels of HDL or "good" cholesterol,
lower high blood pressure,
help improve body composition by burning fat,
promote healthy blood sugar levels,
promote bone density, boost the immune system,
improve mood and reduce the chance of depression.
Vitamins and Minerals, Fibre,Water,
Essential Amino Acids, Essential Fatty Acids,
Essential Saccharides/Carbohydrates,
Antioxidants, Exercise,
Non-toxic Environmen.

LIFT Skin Care

Discover skin care products and see how naturally beautiful your skin can be.

What is the scientists passion about our skin?

Helping you look great, every day, is what we're all about. We know that when you look your best, you also feel your best. That's why we've created products that combine the finest natural ingredients in the world with the most advanced skin care technologies—to keep you beautiful, younger looking and radiant.Created from global technologies and natural, botanical ingredients, our unique and advanced formulas bring out your natural radiance.

What Is the Skin Care System?

The skin care system includes five skin care products—four for the face and one for the body— with proprietary formulas containing numerous natural ingredients to help maintain healthy-looking skin and help fight the signs of aging. The good skin care system contains different botanical ingredients, including extracts and oils from olive fruit, olive leaf, sunflower seed, oat kernel, alfalfa, myrtle leaf, lavender, nutmeg, coconut and ginger. The good system was formulated for the skin care needs of people with all skin types.

Each product in the skin care system contains proprietary blend—a unique combination of minerals and Saccharides that are important for helping maintain healthy, younger-looking skin. The blend is composed of Saccharides from aloe vera leaf juice powder, galactoarabinan and trehalose, along with the mineral-rich clay montmorillonite. The products have extended the use of Saccharides into the skin care system.

How Does the good Skin Care System Work?

The skin is the body's first line of defense and one of the first things people notice when they meet a person face-to-face. The skin can be easily

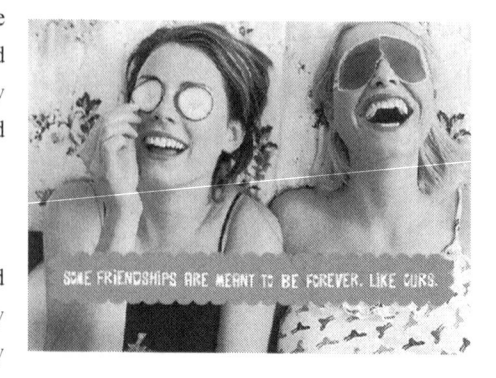

AVERAGE WEIGHT (% dry weight)

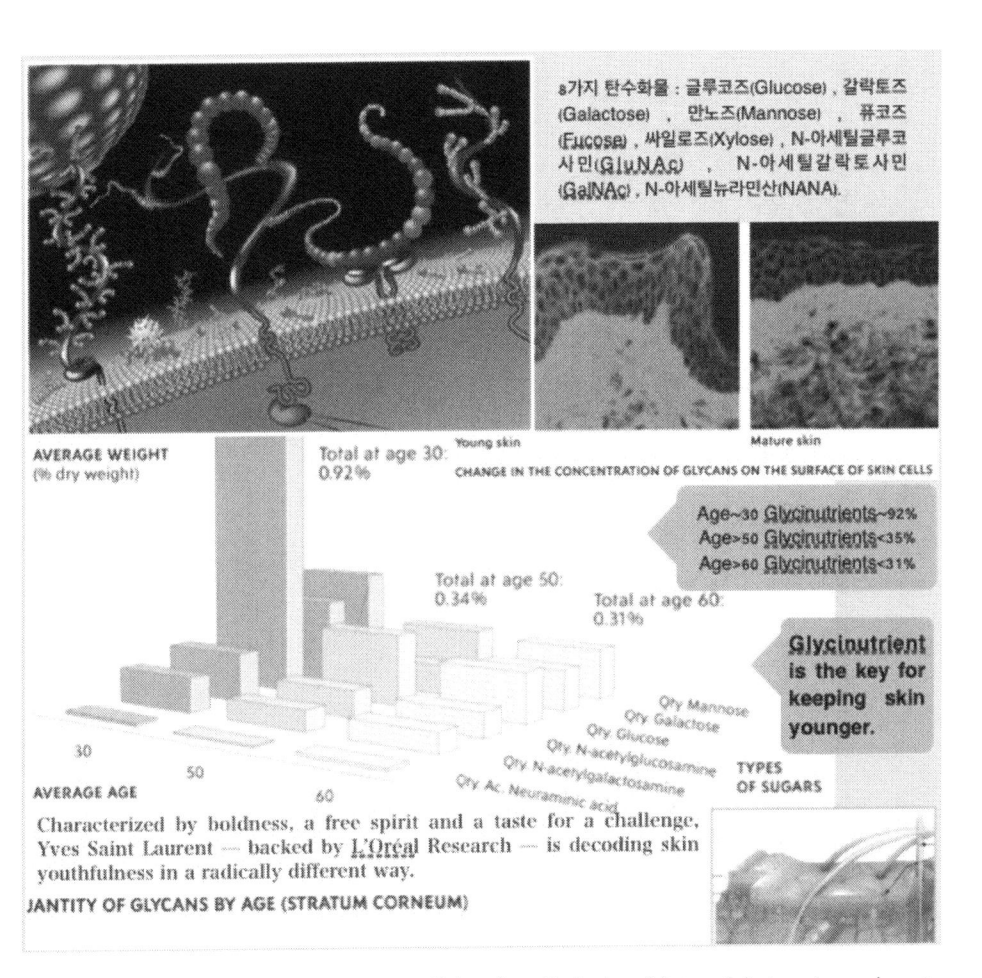

Total at age 30: 0.92% Young skin   Mature skin
CHANGE IN THE CONCENTRATION OF GLYCANS ON THE SURFACE OF SKIN CELLS

8가지 탄수화물 : 글루코즈(Glucose), 갈락토즈(Galactose), 만노즈(Mannose), 퓨코즈(Fucose), 싸일로즈(Xylose), N-아세틸글루코사민(GluNAc), N-아세틸갈락토사민(GalNAc), N-아세틸뉴라민산(NANA).

Age~30 Glycinutrients~92%
Age>50 Glycinutrients<35%
Age>60 Glycinutrients<31%

Total at age 50: 0.34%
Total at age 60: 0.31%

Glycinutrient is the key for keeping skin younger.

Qty Mannose
Qty Galactose
Qty Glucose
Qty N-acetylglucosamine
Qty N-acetylgalactosamine
Qty Ac. Neuraminic acid

AVERAGE AGE   30   50   60   TYPES OF SUGARS

Characterized by boldness, a free spirit and a taste for a challenge, Yves Saint Laurent — backed by L'Oréal Research — is decoding skin youthfulness in a radically different way.

JANTITY OF GLYCANS BY AGE (STRATUM CORNEUM)

damaged by both external factors (e.g., sunlight, air pollution) and internal factors (e.g., cigarette smoke, nutrient-deficient diets). These factors can lead to aging of the skin, dullness and the appearance of fine lines and wrinkles. The best solution to avoid aging of the skin is to stay away from these free-radical producers, use sun protection and eat a healthy diet. However, the use of topical antioxidants and natural moisturizers, such as those found in the good skin care products, can help protect the skin from free radicals and minimize signs of aging.

Why does our skin dry out?

It's the same every year. As the temperature outdoors drops, the air becomes dryer. And biting winds of even 5 mph can cause skin to flake. Indoors isn't much better: Heaters are usually running, which further de-moisturizes the air. Additionally, to keep cold and flu germs at bay, we tend to wash our hands more often, which depletes the skin's natural oils and causes further dryness. Some medications can dry out skin even more. Add in the fact that our skin isn't as young as it used to be, and it's easy to see how these factors combine to make once-lovely skin appear rough and dry. But before you throw up your scratchy hands in despair, there are three simple tips anyone can use to combat the signs of aging and skin dryness.

1. Stay hydrated

This time of year, perhaps more than any other, it's important to drink lots of water. While recommendations vary, in general, if you drink at least eight 8-oz glasses of water every day, it will go a long way toward not only helping your skin stay supple and younger-looking, but also supporting your overall health. Water is just plain good for you!

2. Feed your body what it needs

When we give our bodies proper nutrition—from whole foods, nutrients from nature—our bodies respond by performing at their best. Which means that every cell within them functions optimally, including skin cells! Don't forget to include plenty of omega-3-rich foods in your diet to help fortify the skin's natural oil-retaining barriers.

3. Show your skin some love

Make sure you have a good moisturizer, like the Aloe Body Creme with Saccharides. After bathing or showering, gently pat yourself dry; then apply the lotion generously to help lock in moisture. Don't forget to moisturize dry, cracked heels and rough elbows! Reapply the lotion, gel or cream to exposed areas like your hands throughout the day, especially after washing them.

Bonus tips:

Speaking of your hands, be sure to wash them gently. Use warm water, not hot. Remember that hand sanitizers typically contain about 60% alcohol, which can further dry skin, so you might want to opt for gentle, non-drying soap and water whenever possible. Consider wearing gloves for projects that involve cleaning products, like washing dishes. (One way to think about it is, "Don't let your hands come into contact with anything you wouldn't put on your face, like dishwashing liquid.") And finally, sleep with cotton gloves on at night, after applying a moisturizer, to help your hands stay soft and supple.

With these tips in hand, here's hoping you have a gentle, supple touch all year long!

What You Should Know about Skin Care Product Safety?

Do you ever wonder about the safety of your skin care products? Looking at the ingredient labels on many facial cleansers, moisturizers and body lotions can leave one wondering, "What in the world are most of these things?" and "Is it safe for me to be applying these ingredients to my skin every day?" Currently, it can be difficult for the average consumer to find answers to these questions, which is why the topic of today's blog post is: Skin Care Product Safety—What You Should Know.

Where can you learn more about skin care ingredient safety?

The toxicity of product ingredients is examined almost exclusively by the Cosmetic Ingredient Review (CIR) Expert Panel, an independent committee of scientists and physicians that thoroughly reviews and assesses the safety of ingredients used in cosmetics in the U.S. You can visit www.cir-safety.org to access safety information compiled by CIR. Additional reliable ingredient safety information can also be found on www.cosmeticsinfo.org, a website sponsored by the Personal Care Products Council (PCPC), the leading national trade association representing the global cosmetic and personal care products industry. It is important to note that the safety of many new skin care ingredients has not yet been assessed by CIR.

What do cosmetic companies do to ensure product safety?

Skin care product formulators first work closely with ingredient manufacturers to make certain that they have the most comprehensive and up-to-date ingredient safety information. Following a thorough review of the safety of each ingredient in a formulation, the finished product is subjected to a number of clinical safety tests for adverse reactions such as skin allergy or skin and eye irritations. These tests are performed by scientists who are specially trained in evaluating skin care safety. Once the product is brought to the marketplace, reputable skin care companies continue safety monitoring of consumer experience to help identify any potential safety issues related to their products.

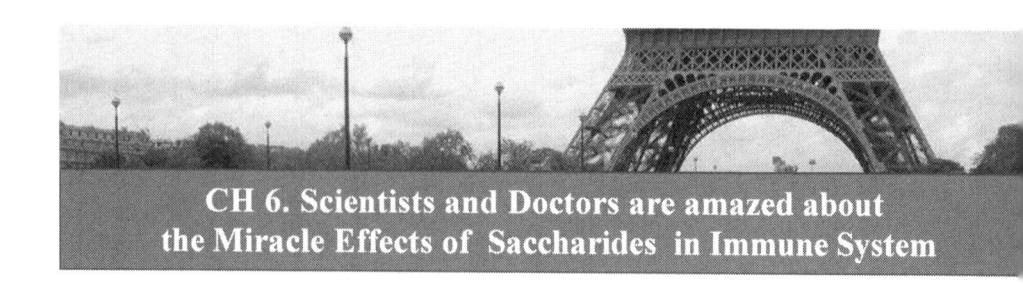

CH 6. Scientists and Doctors are amazed about the Miracle Effects of Saccharides in Immune System

EMERGING TECHNOLOGIE THAT WILL CHANGE THE WORLD

The first on the list is Glycomics. The study of Saccharides is the "EMERGING TECHNOLOGIE THAT WILL CHANGE THE WORLD".

Dr. John Rollins, Former Howard Medical School Professor and U.S. Patent and Trademark Officer calls Saccharides , "One of the most important health discoveries of the 21st Century...I believe that the overall immune supporting potential of Saccharides represents the best integrative health strategy that science has to offer. "

The Science research team presented research showing that these sugars are, in fact digested by colonic bacteria inside the body at the Scripps Center for Innovative Medicine. The Science research team won 1st place that year for their presentation about Saccharides in 2007.

At the 9th Jetter Glycobiology and Medical Symposium held in 2009, there were 33 presentations allowed from the international community of glycobiology researchers.

The first was presented by Dr. Rob Sinnott, he presentation showed data indicating that Saccharides powder has beneficial effects on specific genes that help modulate the immune system.

The second presentation showed an open label human dosing study conducted by St. George's University of London that evaluated the safety and glycosylation effects of Saccharides supplementation. Science research development organization now had the scientific proof that Saccharides supplementation positively influences cell surface sugar structures (glycoproteins), which play a critical role in cell-to-cell communication, proper immune function and optimal health.

In 2009 and 2011, Saccharides supplementation educational website was the recipient of a Web Health Merit Award.

McGraw-Hill Illustrate in Harper's medical textbook for biochemistry that Saccharides supplementation had been sold last year of more than $400 million.

Honoring the 100th anniversary of the vitamin in 2012, Rep. Frank Pallone (D-N.J.) recently entered into the U.S. House of Representatives' Congressional Record remarks recognizing this special milestone. The science research team of Saccharides presented their article in this meeting.

The term "Saccharides " has become the latest buzzword in the food supplements arena. The science of glycobiology , the study of monosaccharides in relation to human health and disease, has remained a complex field addressed primarily within the domain of scientists, clinicians and health researchers.

wikipedia.

What did Scientists & Doctors discover?

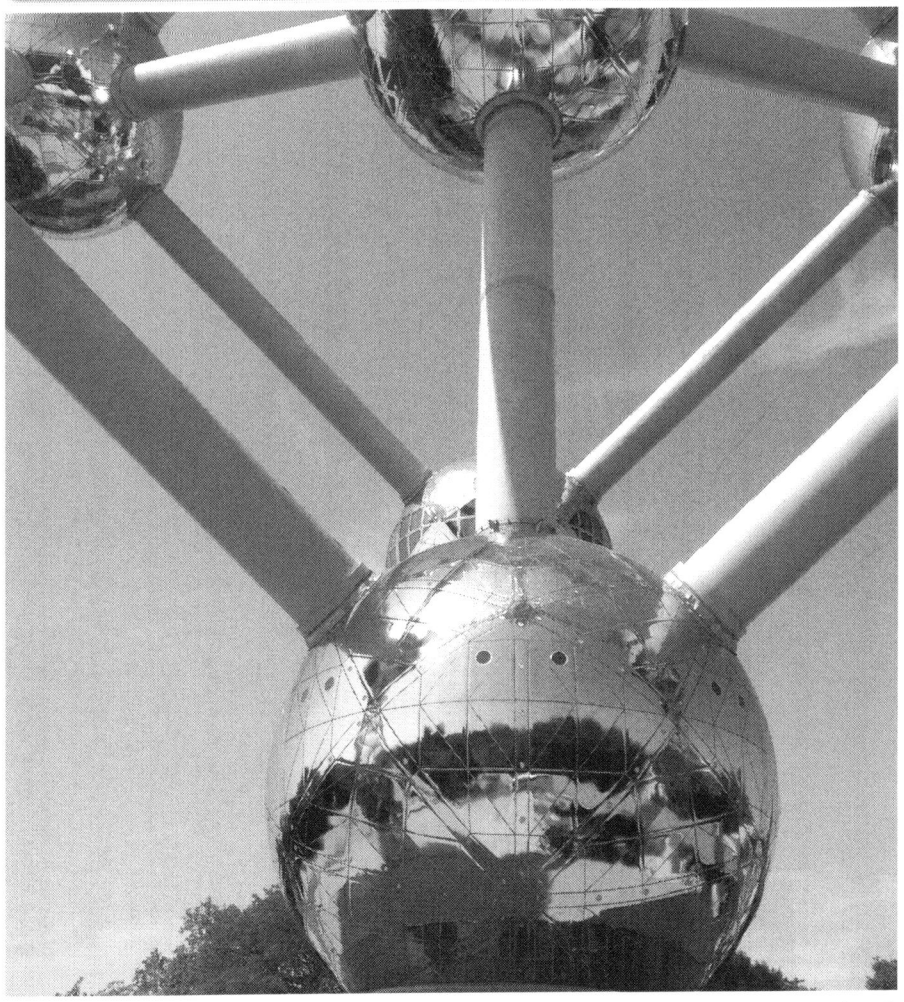

The more doctors learn about Saccharides, the more excited they become about their long-term fundamental health benefits.

The more doctors learn about Saccharides, the more excited they become about their long-term fundamental health benefits. Now, with this new book, the breakthroughs in the study of Saccharides are available to everyone. Whether your goal is to prevent disease, live longer and better, or treat a serious illness that has eluded conventional medicine, Sugars That Heal is your essential guide to complete health.

MIRACLE SUGARS: Scientists have recently discovered that our modern diet is missing some very vital nutrients, and surprisingly enough, these missing nutrients are sugars. After years of research, author Rita Elkins has come to the conclusion that the lack of these invaluable sugars in our diet is a major reason for most of today's diseases, even cancer, diabetes, and auto-immune disorders like rheumatoid arthritis, fibromyalgia, and chronic fatigue syndrome.

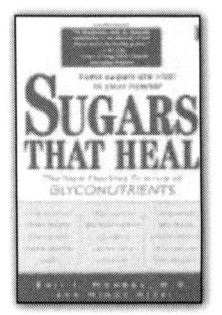

Putting the terms "sugar" and "health" together seems almost like a paradox, but emerging evidence shows that certain types of sugars- commonly called saccharides or Saccharides-are responsible for fighting off disease and maintaining overall health. In MIRACLE SUGARS, author Rita Elkins explains how essential sugars are at the core of our cells' ability to communicate and cooperate in the maintenance and balance of our bodies. The book outlines how these essential saccharides, which are found naturally in food and in available supplements, can fight infection, enhance immune function and battle an impressive variety of health disorders. These sugars have been shown to reverse autoimmune disorders and diabetes, ease allergy symptoms, lower risk of heart disease, and improve overall function of the body's immune processes. Infections respond well to use of saccharides, as do symptoms of fibromyalgia, chronic fatigue and lupus. ven cancer patients have found Saccharides to enhance traditional treatments while lessening their side effects. Saccharides can provide a world of benefits when it comes to your health.

Physician's Management Magazine called the Company the clear leader in the field of nutraceuticals and went on to urge doctors to get involved with the company!

Sugars That Heal: As medical doctor hand scientific researcher Emil Mondoa explains, these essential sugars, known as saccharides, are the basis of multicellular intelligence,the ability of cells to communicate, cohere, and work together to keep us healthy and balanced. Even tiny amounts of these sugars or lack of them have profound effects. In test after test conducted at leading institutes around the world, saccharides have been shown to lower cholesterol, increase lean muscle mass, decrease body fat, accelerate wound healing, ease allergy symptoms, and allay autoimmune diseases such as arthritis, psoriasis, and diabetes. Bacterial infections, including the recurrent ear infections that plague toddlers, often respond remarkably to saccharides, as do many viruses from the common cold to the flu, from herpes to HIV. The debilitating symptoms of chronic fatigue syndrome, fibromyalgia, and Gulf War syndrome frequently abate after adding saccharides. And, for cancer patients, saccharides mitigate the toxic effects of radiation and chemotherapy while augmenting their cancer-killing effects, resulting in prolonged survival and improved quality of life.

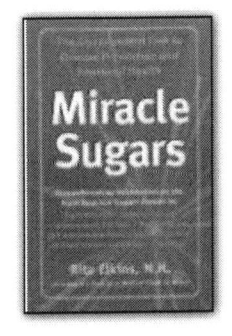

"Sugars that heal" it sounds like a contradiction in terms, but it's the key to one of the most important breakthroughs in recent medical science. We've all been bombarded with warnings about the evils of consuming too much sugar. But, in fact, for our bodies to function properly, we need small amounts of essential sugars, only two of which glucose and galactose are commonly found in our limited, overprocessed diets. When all sugars are available, the health benefits can be breathtaking: Individuals regain their ability to fight disease, reactivate their immune systems, and are able to ward off infection. Based on cutting-edge research in the rapidly evolving science of Saccharides, Sugars That Heal is an exciting new approach to health and disease prevention.

Sugars That Heal offers a revolutionary new health plan based on the science of Saccharides-- foods that contain saccharides. It gives authoritative guidance for getting all saccharides conveniently into your diet through supplements and readily available foods, as well as **Natural Muscle magazine** :"How To Thrive on an Ailing Planet - Glycoproteins." by Spice Williams-Crosby (July '99). This article discussed how to overcome the deficiencies in our modern-day diet.

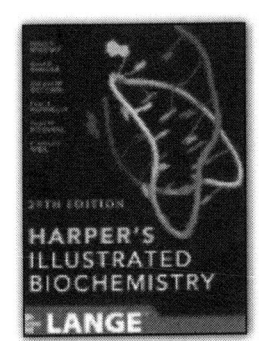

Harpers Biochemistry is the definitive reference for medical students and contains the latest information in the field of Biochemistry. Chapter 56, entitled Glycoproteins is devoted to glycoscience. This textbook has been educating healthcare professionals about Saccharides and their role in health and healing since 1996. According to Harper's Biochemistry textbook, only 2 or 3 of the necessary 8 Saccharides are commonly found in our diet.

Scientific American ~ July 2002.

"Sweet Medicine: Building Better Drugs from Sugars." Sugars play critical roles in many cellular functions and in disease. Study of those activities lags behind research into genes and proteins but is beginning to heat up. The discoveries promise to yield a new generation of drug therapies.

Scientific American

~ September-October 2003. "The Sweet Science of Glycobiology" Complex carbohydrates, molecules that are particularly important for communication among cells, are coming under systematic study.

Carbohydrates are indispensable to life on Earth. In their simplest form, they serve as a primary energy source for sustaining life. For the most part, however, carbohydrates exist not as simple sugars but as complex molecular conjugates, or glycans. Glycans come in many shapes and sizes, from linear chains (polysaccharides) to highly branched molecules bristling with antennae-like arms. And although proteins and nucleic acids such as DNA have traditionally attracted far more scientific attention, glycans are also key to life. They are ubiquitous in nature, forming the intricate sugar coat that surrounds the cells of virtually every organism and occupying the spaces between these cells. As part of this so-called extracellular matrix, glycans, with their diverse chemical structures, play a crucial role in transmitting important biochemical signals into and between cells. In this way, these sugars guide the cellular communication that is essential for normal cell and tissue development and physiological function.

Karate magazine featured an interview with Dr. Bob Ward (former strength and conditioning coach for the Dallas Cowboys) in which he recommended Saccharides because of "their ability to enhance athletic performance better than anything else on the market."

Acta Anatomica ~ Glycosciences, Issue 161/1-April 1998

International Journal of Anatomy, Embryology and Cell Biology. The Acta Anatomica is a highly respected scientific journal, featuring our scientific breakthrough. The article explains the unsurpassed coding capacity of the 8 Saccharides that make up our discovery and states: "Glycosylation is the most common form of protein and lipid modification but its biological significance has long been underestimated. The last decade, however, has witnessed the rapid emergence of the concept of the sugar code of biological information. Monosaccharides represent an alphabet of biological information similar to amino acids and nucleic acids but with unsurpassed coding capacity."

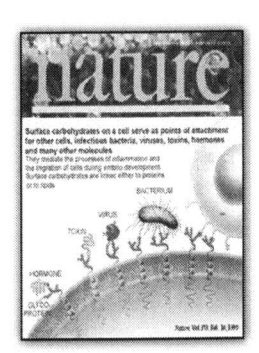

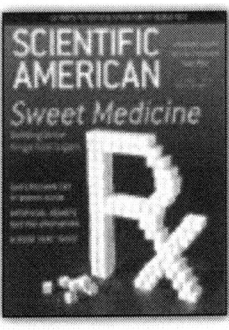

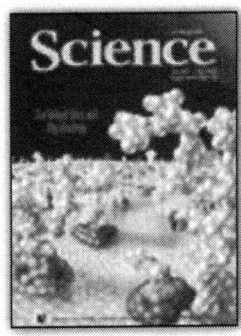

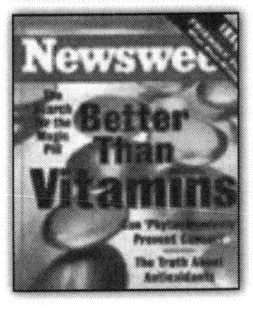

Newsweek (April 25, 1994) featured a story that talked about the power of the same substances in Saccharides to "kill and necrose cancer in the human cell"

The Department of Nutrition and Food Sciences at Texas Woman's University (TWU*) are developing and implementing collaborative endeavors that will enhance the public's knowledge about health and nutrition. On April 15, 2011, Professor Francesco Marotta**, MD, PhD, gave a lecture to TWU Nutrition and Food Sciences students titled "Clinical Options and Applications for Genetic Testing in Modern Nutritional Strategies."

Science Magazine, Special Issue ~ Carbohydrates & Glycobiology, March 23, 2001. A publication of Stanford University for the American Association for the Advancement of Science, Science Magazine dedicated an entire 200-page magazine issue to educating the science and medical community about Saccharides, Glycobiology and Glycoscience.

Physician's Desk Reference (PDR) for Nonprescription Drugs and Dietary Supplements lists only scientifically validated (peer reviewed) products and is distributed to over 300,000 physicians each year. Our company's Saccharide products are listed in this book by name. **Eclipse: Miracle** in South Dallas Nov-Dec, 2001.

Special 'sugars' change the academic performance of some Dallas school children who many had given up on.

The Healing Power of 8 Sugars: An Amazing Breakthrough in Nutrition, Sciences and Medicine
Allan C. Somersall (Editor)
Publication Date: May 2005
Doctors from different fields combine their varied perspectives and diverse experiences to reveal the increasing weight of clinical evidence for the therapeutic benefits of Saccharides (the 8-essential sugars the body needs) in a wide range of medical conditions.

Change mind, change live.

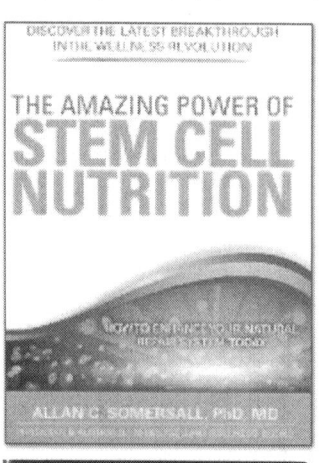

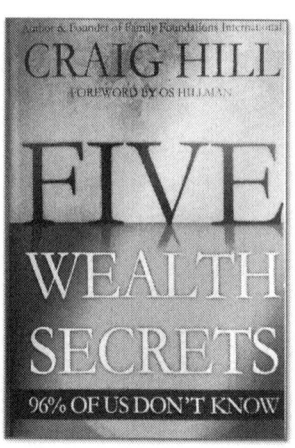

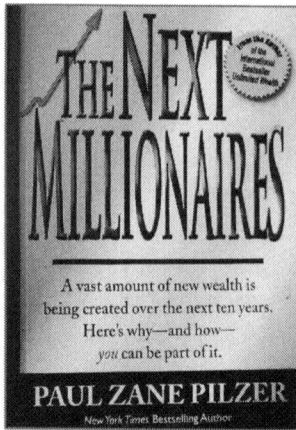

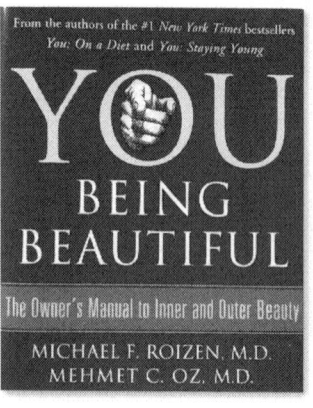

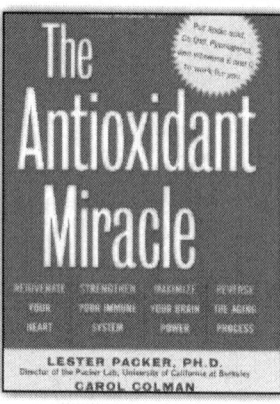

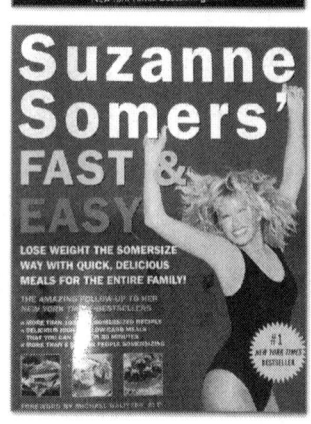

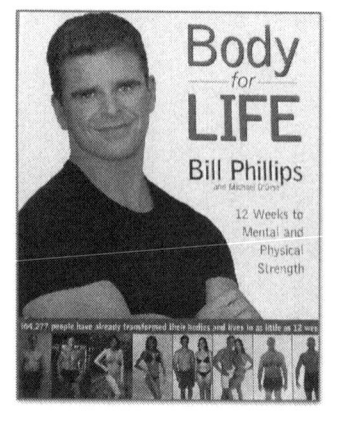

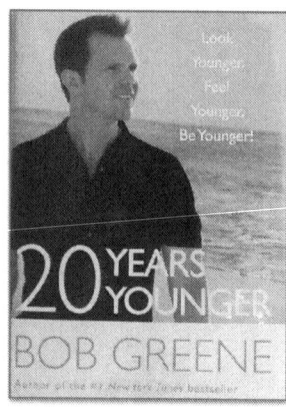

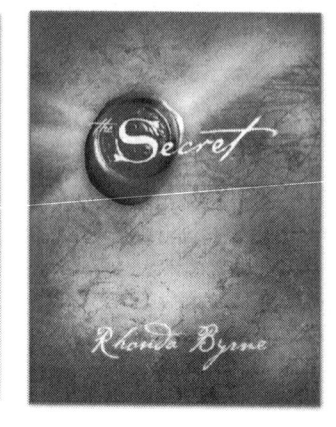

55

Printed in Great Britain
by Amazon